LITTLE EARTHQUAKES

LITTLE EARTHQUAKES

A MEMOIR

SARAH MANDEL

HARPER

An Imprint of HarperCollins*Publishers*

LITTLE EARTHQUAKES. Copyright © 2023 by Sarah Mandel. All rights reserved. Printed in the United States of America. No part of this book may be used or reproduced in any manner whatsoever without written permission except in the case of brief quotations embodied in critical articles and reviews. For information, address HarperCollins Publishers, 195 Broadway, New York, NY 10007.

HarperCollins books may be purchased for educational, business, or sales promotional use. For information, please email the Special Markets Department at SP-sales@harpercollins.com.

FIRST EDITION

Designed by Leah Carlson-Stanisic

Library of Congress Cataloging-in-Publication Data has been applied for.

ISBN 978-0-06-327091-6

23 24 25 26 27 LBC 5 4 3 2 1

For Sophie and Siena—I love you both *unerasable*.

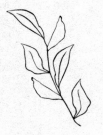

with surprising gaiety I am saying thank you as I
remember who I am, a woman learning to praise
something as small as dandelion petals floating on the
steaming surface of this bowl of vegetable soup,
my happy, savoring tongue.

—Jeanne Lohmann, "To Say Nothing but Thank You"

CONTENTS

PART II BETRAYAL

PART III DISSOCIATION

PART IV WAKING

PART V INTEGRATION

INTRODUCTION

Staring at my bedroom ceiling was the most I was able to do some days. Yet I can tell you nothing about what my surroundings looked like: I do not know if there were any cracks in the molding or if a chip of the pale blue paint was missing, revealing the darker-hue of concrete below. On one occasion, I snapped out of this haze, looked at my clock, and saw that three hours had passed. I had been "awake," but nothing, absolutely nothing, had happened. Not a single thought had entered my mind. I had not moved even a pinkie toe. It was as if I had been in a suspended state of consciousness, separate from myself, time, and space.

Only six months prior, my husband and I had been sitting at our dining table on a Sunday evening, feeling accomplished after putting our four-year-old daughter down to sleep. With all of Manhattan twinkling outside our twentieth-floor windows, Derek, his blue-gray eyes also sparkling, looked at me and said, "Wow, we are so lucky." I wholeheartedly agreed. There was a vibrancy to our lives in that early fall of 2017: we were all healthy; Derek and I worked in our dream jobs, me as a clinical psychologist, he in strategy and operations at a major tech company; we were in constant awe of our little girl, Sophie; and I was far enough along in my second pregnancy that we were able to safely envision the adventure of adding another little person to our growing family.

The next morning, after a routine medical examination that was meant to be a pit stop en route to work, I was told that, in all likelihood, I had a fatal form of cancer. The lump in my breast, which both my OBGYN and I believed indicated that my body was getting ready to feed my soon-to-be-born baby, was not a milk duct after all. Later that week I was officially diagnosed with breast cancer, which, soon thereafter, was categorized as Stage IV. The cancer had metastasized and spread throughout my body.

Suddenly, at thirty-six years old and in my third trimester of my second pregnancy, I became a member of a statistical group for whom there is a 73 percent chance of dying within five years.[1] Life as I knew it halted abruptly: my work as a therapist, playdates, walks through Central Park, and trips to the Bronx Zoo were replaced with treatment infusions and inpatient hospital stays. When not receiving oncology-related treatments, I was mostly confined to my bed, where Sophie and my newborn baby, Siena, were brought to me for snuggles and stories. Any attempt to leave my bedroom required my using a walker to hold me steady, as my bones had been eaten away by cancer lesions. My body was literally breaking down and falling apart.

But in early January 2018—after only three months of cancer treatment—I was categorized into another statistically rare group: there was no longer evidence of the disease in my body, a status known as NED. This extraordinary treatment outcome occurs in only 5.5 percent of metastatic breast cancer patients.[2] My loving family and friends were overjoyed by the miraculous news. But the whiplash from living to dying to possibly living again resulted in a state of perpetual bewilderment. I could make no sense of the facts that were my life. *What in the hell had just happened?*

I had encountered this overwhelming sense of confusion and shock in my clinical psychology practice. As a specialist in trauma therapy, I had more than twenty years of experience working or volunteering with traumatized populations and patients. But now I had a trauma of my own.

According to the fifth edition of *The Diagnostic and Statistical Manual of Mental Disorders (DSM-V)*, psychological trauma involves an "exposure to actual or threatened death, serious injury, or sexual violence."[3] Typically, the reaction to threat almost instantaneously activates the body's sympathetic nervous system, also referred to as the "fight-or-flight" response. When you perceive a threat (either real or imagined), your sensory system relays a message to your brain, specifically the cerebral cortex (responsible for rational thought), which thereafter sends an alarm to the amygdala (a brain structure involved in emotion processing). Fight-or-flight is a hardwired mechanism present in all mammals during which the body reacts to danger by fighting the threat or escaping to safety. This involuntary response results in a formidable surge of energy that serves us well in times of peril.[4]

For example, if you accidentally place your hand on a hot stove, pain sensory neurons in your brain send off a message to the spinal cord and then specific brain regions regarding the location and intensity of the burn.[5] This automatic pain response results in you swiftly removing that hand from the source of injury within a half a second from initial contact. Without the pain signaling, you would leave your palm on that burning stove and suffer a severe skin wound. Pain is critical to our safety.

Like pain, fear is also adaptive and potentially lifesaving.[6] Yet despite its adaptiveness, fight-or-flight may be an insufficient response in traumatizing circumstances, such as when a child is subjected to sexual abuse, a soldier witnesses an atrocity at war, or an adult is involved in a near-fatal car crash.

In these highly traumatic situations, the fight-or-flight system is activated, but the ordinarily protective body reactions are rendered inadequate. Trapped in a horrifying circumstance, a profound sense of helplessness and abject terror ensues. The mind and body scream out to fight or escape—but to no avail. Instead, we experience a loss of faith in the notion of safety in our bodies, and perhaps a generalized fear of the world at large.[7] When escape is impossible, the mind and body surrender into a frozen state of collapse—a response of the sympathetic nervous system known as "freeze." A constellation of posttraumatic stress symptoms, including a chronically aroused state that intends to protect from future threat, may become entrenched in a person's new way of living.[8]

This was the frozen posture I found myself in as I lay motionless in bed, even though the threat of cancer had eased.

I learned early on in my clinical training that trauma is far more common than we may think at first blush. Prevalence research suggests that 89.7 percent of the U.S. population will experience a *DSM-V*-defined traumatic event during their lifetime.[9] Yet a significant stigma is still associated with mental health conditions, and traumatic experiences, in particular. Our cultural norms dictate that we shouldn't talk about the gruesome, the depressing, or the terrifying—whether it's abuse, neglect, or the natural process of death and grieving.

So often, these cruel human experiences land deep within the bodies and minds of trauma sufferers, who feel caged in their silence. Trauma can tear apart a person's sense of safety, connection to self and others, and meaning in life. And for many, their trauma history feels like an open wound that will never heal over.

Paradoxically, the more we avoid or attempt to quiet traumatic memories and related thoughts, the more they rear their heads to haunt us. Our brains don't play along with our best efforts at avoidance.[10] According to clinical psychology research, recovery from posttraumatic stress symptoms is due to *habituation*—the gradual exposure to distressing trauma memories results in their eventually losing their initial, often debilitating, emotional impact.[11] We begin to melt from our frozen state, and return to our sensing, feeling, and thinking selves.

Many of my patients have struggled with posttraumatic stress disorder (PTSD) symptoms related to childhood physical, sexual, or emotional abuse; or perhaps they witnessed violence or were a recent victim of assault. At the start of therapy, I assure my patients that they will dictate the pace of treatment; I am here to travel alongside them, but they are in the driver's seat. This safety-increasing intervention is essential for those who have experienced the profound helplessness of a freeze state.

After reviewing emotional, cognitive, and interpersonal coping skills, my patients and I delve into the narrative work. I give my patients permission to look at their scary thoughts and to learn, over time, that thoughts can't actually hurt them. Together we revisit and organize their memories and then construct a narrative around their trauma so that the once-fragmented story ultimately has a beginning, middle, and end. Through their narrative work, my patients are able to commit their histories to the past, embrace life in the present, and plan for the future.

After days on end of lying in bed and casting my eyes at that ceiling, I started to feel afraid. I was healing physically from the cancer. But would I be stuck in this psychological state of dissociation forever? Was this what the rest of my life was going to be like, mindlessly staring at a wall? I was technically alive, with a steady beating pulse, but I felt as if I had flatlined. I experienced none of the peaks and valleys of emotional experience that typically punctuate daily living. I was shrouded in a veneer of dulled detachment.

I was desperate to wake myself up. Then the psychologist in me started to wonder: Maybe the act of writing could rouse my seemingly dormant brain cells? As I mulled over the possibility, I realized that there were parts of my trauma—the diagnosis, cancer treatment, and its aftermath—that I had not been able to face or make sense of through language. Perhaps, I thought, I could experiment with trauma narrative therapy for *myself* and discover whether treatments I have provided to my patients could also be of use to me. Maybe narrative therapy could help me start to feel again?

During the initial cancer-crisis days, I knew that my lab and body scan reports were just a few clicks away on my medical center's online "portal," but I purposely avoided information about my condition. Since it was too frightening to face the details (the likelihood of my dying in five years, for example), I operated under the assumption that my doctors would curate the medical information so that I would be made aware of the necessary facts only. It wasn't until after I decided to write my trauma narrative that I was able to study my cancer medical reports, google the bewildering Latin phrases and terminology, and read the randomized controlled trial results about my type of cancer treatment. Scrolling down my medical report pdfs, I was confronted with the hard facts that lacked any of the human sugarcoating my doctors provided. Each startling word—*carcinoma, extensive lytic lesions, calcification, cortical destruction*—like a punch to my gut.

As I played medical detective, I also became a psychological detective, gathering the pieces of a surreal set of truths. I searched through emails I'd sent to friends and family and studied photographs from the previous eight months: me just minutes after giving birth to my second baby; leaning on my walker to hold my body upright while visiting my four-year-old's school bake sale; cozying up with my mother under mounds of the white, heated hospital blankets in the cancer center's waiting room. At the outset of my writing, my memories and the collected data resembled a disassembled puzzle in a chaotic heap. But I felt comfort in knowing that I was starting the important work of revisiting my past.

Shedding my doctor identity, I assumed the role of psychology patient. Though clearly an unorthodox treatment plan ("therapist heal thyself" is typically not recommended!), I knew that my personal psychotherapist was at the ready if my writing proved to be emotionally unbearable. I hoped that by slowly and compassionately revisiting my trauma memories and organizing them on paper, I could find new understanding and reengage with my emotional repertoire.

And, dear reader, it worked. Word by word, my story broke free from the haze of my traumatized mind.

My writing, in combination with safely moving my once-immobile body, were the catalysts that roused my brain from its foggy, chemo-ridden, trauma-dissociated state. Writing about myself required organizational, creative, and problem-solving cognitive faculties. I presumed that many of my brain cells had not survived the chemotherapy assault and had atrophied and died. Perhaps, through my writing, I was exercising my brain's potential to create new neurons—that very hopeful neurological process known as neurogenesis.[12] I also imagined that my inactive brain neurons were like the bits of glittery-white settled at the base of a snow globe, and that my writing shook them up as, once again, they learned to whirl in all directions.

I was determined to remember my trauma, to put it down somewhere outside of myself—and what I found was this act of writing provided significant emotional relief. While I was living through the crisis days, life had an unreal quality to it. But bringing words to that haziness helped me emerge from the dissociative fog and gain clarity. Writing became a source of validation—my experience was real, those words upon the page were the story of my life. My storytelling was also empowering; I could take the helm in managing my memories and create meaning from them. And, ultimately, I realized that these memories were an important part of me, but they were not *all* of me.

In the summer of 2020, there were still days when I stared out, blankly—perhaps recovering after a recent infusion and too fatigued to read, talk, or watch a TV show. But I no longer felt traumatically triggered as I lay in bed. I knew that the beach was just steps away from the seaside home where we were staying, and that soon enough I would have the strength to walk along the uneven pebbly shore, attempt to skip rocks along the surface of the bay, and swim out into the vast blueness of the water and sky.

When my energy returned, I gathered up my children and their pink, green, and blue sandcastle-building pails, and we tumbled down the grassy hill to the water's edge. We listened to the rush of the bay. We searched for hermit crabs and shimmery, "magic" rocks. I was surrounded by smiling little faces, the sweet sound of my girls' giggles and full-bellied laughter, and the invigorating breeze of fresh ocean air.

Up until a few years ago, I had always been afraid of the sea and the unknown beneath the surface—possible critters with pinchers or that sinking feeling of mushy wet sludge under my bare feet, not knowing what that gooey *stuff* is. Earlier in my life, embarrassing as it is to admit, I also steered clear of swimming to avoid having my eyeliner run. Once we had our first child, Derek was designated the "play in the water" parent, as fear and vanity kept me glued to the beach or lounge chair. I took in the beauty of the view, and that was just fine with me.

It took cancer to finally call me into the ocean. I typically don't wear makeup anymore, and certainly wouldn't wear any on a beach day—so that earlier fear of raccoon eyes is moot. I've now made a promise to myself that if I'm visiting a body of water and the temperature is reasonable, I've got to go in. Once I submerge my body, my sensory system takes over and is amplified 1,000,000 percent. I feel the shock of the cold on my skin, but then I acclimate. I notice the muffled silence below the surface as I dive, and the feeling of the ocean gently holding me as I float back to meet the sky. I play, I explore, and I feel free.

A SPECIAL NOTE TO READERS

My story is one of sickness, trauma, unpredictability, and pain; but, most of all, it is a story of healing. I move through the stages of trauma, and I invite you to travel through them with me. Let your body and mind be your guide and pace yourself as you enter my world. At its most intense moments, hold close the knowledge that this is a story of hope and recovery. We will get there together, I promise.

If you are struggling with trauma-related or other distressing mental health symptoms, please reach out to a care provider. You will find a list of resources in the appendix of this book, including how to locate a psychotherapist. You do not need to struggle on your own. Help is available, and recovery can be your story, too.

PART I

SURVIVAL

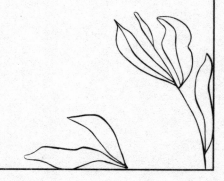

1

A DIFFERENT PREGNANCY

My husband and I sat with my therapist in her Manhattan office, discussing the postpartum plan. Midway through my pregnancy, in the early summer of 2017, I was on a mission to avoid the depression that had engulfed me after the birth of my first little girl. I was astonished that on day two of being a mom the nurses had handed me a real live person, allowed us to leave the hospital with her, and actually expected us to know how to care for this newborn, who turned upside down everything we knew about how we lived our adult, independent lives. Those first few weeks, in particular, were surreal. Sleeping-sort-of during the day as our baby napped, and up all night. Trying to make it outside for fresh air during the daylight, to look at the world, still turning.

When we made it out of our apartment, maybe before 2:00 P.M. if we were lucky (assembling the diaper bag of life-supporting necessities while operating on mere pockets of interrupted sleep was an exercise in absurdity), we looked through the slits of our heavy-lidded eyes at everyone on the New York

City streets and said aloud—How are there all of these people, who were once babies? The parade of adults zipping by had all been infants. The floppy-haired boy, joyfully riding his scooter, had been a baby. A cheery-looking woman walked by with *two* children in tow. The guy pushing his toddler in a stroller looked perfectly coiffed, rested, and emotionally stable—we could tick none of those boxes. We were utterly baffled that many grown-ups actually had chosen to have more than one child. How was it that humankind continued to propagate, despite the near torture that comes with caring for a newborn? Our assessment was clear: being a parent is nuts!

In those initial postpartum days, I wasn't lucky enough to know that the light at the end of that initial sleepless tunnel is so bright, so rewarding, it will make your heart feel like it's going to burst. My love for my daughter, Sophie, continued to grow daily. I was intoxicated by the sound of her laughter tickling my eardrum. I marveled at her wide-brown-eyed curiosity or the scrunched-up look of determination on her round, cherubic face. And then, in what seemed like some act of genius, she learned to speak and became an active conversationalist— What would she say next? Motherhood swelled with the privilege and joy I had always hoped it would. The yearning for another child to nuzzle and smell, to get to know and love, to bring into Sophie's world, eclipsed any fears of becoming ill again after delivery.

Almost four years after Sophie's birth, I'd also developed professional expertise in maternal mental health. Based on my own encounters with motherhood and postpartum depression, I felt inspired to expand my therapy offerings to other new parents. I sought out specialized training in perinatal depression, anxiety, and bereavement; facilitated new moms groups; and devoted much of my psychology practice to providing cognitive-behavioral therapy to pregnant and postpartum women. It had become my life's work and passion.

In short, my husband, Derek, and I were armed and ready to keep me well this time around. As part of my personal and professional education, I had read all the books on postpartum depression, including the appropriately titled *What Am I Thinking? Having a Baby after Postpartum Depression*.[1] I had scanned and printed out the book's "Postpartum Pact," which was a four-page checklist meant to be reviewed with one's partner prior to giving birth. Sections included *Here's what I need you to listen for*, followed by warning signs bullet-pointed with empty squares ready for a check mark: *Do I say I just don't feel like myself? Am I expressing feelings of inadequacy, failure, or hopelessness? Am I afraid I will always feel this way?* Derek was invited to join me and my individual psychologist for a one-time therapy session, and I brought the Pact with me to the appointment, always the prepared pupil with my lists and pens at the ready. My therapist helped us review the document together, our fears aired in the safety of her office as Derek and I alternated between holding hands and letting our bent legs lean into each other, together on that gray, firm couch where I had spent countless hours of my life.

"I only worry that she'll have a hard time if something unexpected happens," Derek shared with us, his eyes meeting mine only after finishing his sentence. I thought his words over. Imagining any complications with the health of our soon-to-be-born baby was daunting. What if the baby had a neurodevelopmental disorder? I remembered, with Sophie, anxiously awaiting her first "social smile," which would suggest that her mirror neurons—the brain cells essential for social interaction

and empathy—were functioning normally. I sighed with relief when Sophie gifted me that first magnificent, gummy baby
smile in response to my own. But then there were other fears
about this second pregnancy. What if the baby had some genetic
disorder that had not been identified in utero? Or if there was a
serious complication during the birth? And then the worst fear
of all—what if we lost our baby?

I reassured Derek (and myself) of the unlikelihood of a serious, unanticipated problem. Statistics were on our side that
we would have a healthy baby. With my history of postpartum
depression, *I* was the one who was most in danger of becoming
ill.[2] Knowing my risk, I had planned accordingly. I was now on
an antidepressant medication that would help hold me steady
during the turbulent physical, biological, and hormonal changes
of the postpartum period. I had also done the hard work in therapy to challenge my previous, rigidly held belief that my depression made me a *terrible mother*. Back then, I was convinced
that I was the only new parent struggling with self-doubt, panic,
and crippling shame. But I was wrong: women are particularly
vulnerable to depressive symptoms during and after pregnancy,
and a whopping 15 to 20 percent suffer from postpartum depression.[3, 4] Yet the stigma around the range of psychological
distress associated with motherhood is so thick that new moms
are often invisible in their suffering, pretending to be well when
in fact they feel as if they are shattered into pieces. Like them, I
pretended, too.

My therapist highlighted that "this pregnancy and postpartum period will be different" because we had learned so much
during the four years since the birth of our first child. I no longer viewed early motherhood as a picture-perfect fantasyland,
so I was not at risk of the same steep fall from that unattainable

peak. I was medicated. We arranged for childcare to ensure that I would get much-needed sleep. We had a well-thought-out plan that met my perfectionistic yearnings. I would *not* get sick this time.

My therapist was right: this second pregnancy was already different. When Sophie was in utero, the surge of hormones brought on an almost euphoric state. I felt like I had an orb of positivity radiating from inside me that each week expanded even more, resulting in an ever-present smile across my blissed-out face. I was in awe of my body, its ability to create life, to feel the kicks and jabs of a real person inside me. I was that "glowing" pregnant woman, cherishing the closeness of carrying my baby with me always, hearts beating so close together, all the time. I felt like Mother Earth.

This second pregnancy didn't make me feel so rosy. The tolerable dry-heaving that marked my first trimester with Sophie was replaced with severe nausea and vomiting. I survived on a diet of ginger chews, oyster crackers, and, if it was a good day, some form of carbohydrate sprinkled with melted cheese. I didn't eat any meals for months. My relationship with food comprised tentative, obligatory bites throughout the day. The nausea was so disruptive that it forced my hand, and at only nine weeks I told my bosses that I would have to rearrange my patient schedule to accommodate my pregnancy evening, not morning, sickness. I needed to be home before 7:00 P.M., when I launched into my inevitable nightly puking ritual.

An antivomiting medication took a little of the edge off, but it also put me into a state of near total exhaustion. Luckily the nausea resolved in my second trimester, but what took its place was still not anywhere near a "glow." This second pregnancy felt less magical, more pragmatic. I had a three-year-old and a busy psychology practice. I was simply going through the pregnancy motions.

My body ached—hips, ribs, back—and the prenatal yoga classes and cardio workouts I had continued throughout my first pregnancy became painfully off-limits. I sought out physical and massage therapy in hope of some relief. The chronic soreness, peppered with bouts of shooting pain, remained. The right hip area was especially finicky and at times demanded that I not even place my right foot upon the ground to walk. When I insisted on moving, my hip would protest with a sharp pang.

Though I was burdened by these pregnancy woes, I was most of all excited to meet my little person. It was comforting to know that soon enough I would have my warm, lovable infant in my arms. That my body would find itself back to a place of strength, ability, and pain-free movement. I was okay with the temporary status of my discomfort—because a baby is one hell of a prize to get at the end.

At the five-month mark of my pregnancy, I found a little lump, like a tiny pebble, in my right breast. No reason to get concerned, I told myself: I have a tendency to have lots of body oddities that turn out to be benign, if not bizarre. I was only in my midthirties and in the second trimester with my second pregnancy. I googled *breast lump during pregnancy*. My computer screen filled up with search results that cancer tumors are extremely rare during pregnancy, and that milk duct clogging is quite common. I imagined my body getting ready to feed and nourish my baby, which, according to my weekly pregnancy app update, was the size of a large mango. The lump was likely just another growing round shape I harbored, like two planets in orbit, the primordial beginnings within my own celestial body.

At thirty-three weeks, I noticed that the once-small pebble in my breast had become firm and round, and much larger, like a gumball. During my Friday appointment, I flagged the issue with my OBGYN. She agreed with Google, assuring me that it was likely just a milk duct issue but encouraged me to get it further examined in order to have the duct cleared prior to the birth of my baby. That way, we could hopefully avoid any complications with breastfeeding.

I scheduled the sonogram for Monday and spent much of the next two days following the doctor and Google's at-home care. I took long showers, angling the showerhead and hot water directly onto the spot to "loosen up" the milk. While watching television with Derek, I sat with my left hand down the front of my T-shirt and aggressively massaged the lump in hopes of releasing the clogged milk. My husband thought I was crazy. Isn't this a little excessive? he said. He tolerated my dedication with a mixture of bewilderment and amusement.

On Monday, lump still lumpy, I sat in the waiting room at the radiology office on East Eighty-Fourth Street. A fortysomething-year-old woman sitting across from me talked enthusiastically and loudly into her cell phone, sharing with her friend, and all of us in the waiting room, specifics about her date the prior evening, her recent and outrageous shopping spree, and her sex life. Eye rolls and looks of disbelief filled the room as she went on and on, unaware of her surroundings or simply not caring. I wondered which of the women in the room were anxious about getting scanned after previous cancer scares or perhaps an actual diagnosis.

Once inside the sonogram room, I arranged myself on the reclined examination chair, my belly big and uncooperative. The overhead lights were off as the technician slid the sonogram wand across my breasts. A blurry, gray scale image of my flesh emerged and then disappeared, again and again, on the corresponding computer monitor. I initiated small talk. She told me that the doctor was going to check me as well. It was my first breast sonogram, and all of this appeared routine.

Dr. Berson, a tall, athletic-looking man perhaps in his fifties, entered the room and was both personable and professional. He moved his wand in motions like the infinity symbol over my breasts for several minutes. I started to worry. Are breast sonograms usually this long and detailed?

I remember the darkness of the room when he told me that the sonogram looked suspicious for a malignancy, and that I would need a mammogram and biopsy. Cloaked in shadows, I felt as if I were in some sort of dream, separate from the real world just outside that examination room's door. Dr. Berson said that he would try everything he could to schedule the biopsy for later that day. I became aware of my stilted breathing, reminded myself to inhale and exhale, and tried to steady myself with logic.

But no matter how hard my brain tried, I didn't understand. I kept repeating to myself, I'm thirty-six. I'm pregnant. I have no family history of early-onset cancer or other risk factors. I'm about to go to work to see my patients in an hour. There's been some kind of mistake. I held on to my late grandmother's words that had become a family mantra: *everything will be just fine, dearie.*

In the changing room, the shock and disbelief briefly dispelled by the fluorescent lights, I noticed that I wanted to cry out the word "Mommy." I dug my cell phone out of my purse, called my mom, and told her, "Something's not right. I'm at the breast sonogram appointment—they think the lump looks suspicious." There was a steadiness to her voice and clear loving concern. She was immediately on her way over from her apartment, thankfully only several blocks away, to meet me.

Then I called my husband, who was flying to Phoenix on a business trip. He had left so early for the airport—still in the dark of the early morning as he slipped out of our apartment without waking me or our Sophie, his small, trusty black roller suitcase following him out the door—that I thought he'd have landed by then. When I got no answer, I left him a message, my voice intentionally composed as I said, "Please call me back." I texted. I emailed, "Please call me when you get this." But twenty minutes later he responded, via email, that he was still up in the air. I thought to myself, I can't write that I may have cancer in an email. But I'd scared him already; he knew that something was wrong.

When Dr. Berson told me that he'd arranged to do the biopsy that day and to wait in the examination room for the procedure, I called work and said that there was an emergency and that I couldn't make it into the office. The administrative assistant canceled all of my patients for the day. Since they knew that I was in the third trimester of my pregnancy, I took solace in the fact that they would most likely assume my absence was baby-, and not cancer-, related.

In preparation for the biopsy, I asked Dr. Berson if I could borrow a shirt. He looked at me for a moment, head tilted, trying to parse my strange request. I was wearing the one professional-looking shirt that still fit me and my belly, I said. I'd outgrown all the rest and would have nothing left to wear to my office if I got blood on it. At the time, I still expected I would return to work the next day.

During the biopsy, I chatted with Dr. Berson and, despite

the unusual circumstances, found myself enjoying our conversation. He lived in the same neighborhood where I grew up,
where my parents still reside. We talked Judaism and New York
City schools. I took deep inhalations as I felt each zap in my
breasts and armpits as he collected cells with a vacuum-like
suctioning needle.

Derek, who had just landed in Phoenix, called immediately
following the biopsy. Dr. Berson stepped away from me mo-
mentarily to retrieve and then hand me my phone, knowing
that I needed to take the call. I don't remember much of what
was said. As I sat upright, still topless, stripes of blood started
to trickle down my breasts and round belly. Derek was at the
airport, I managed to comprehend from his words. What was
going on? he asked me. I didn't know. I found myself trying
to protect him, to protect his work trip, to be OK for him and
help him stay calm despite the distance and fear between us.
Meanwhile, Dr. Berson must have been tending to my wounds,
though I don't remember because I was so focused on my call
with Derek. But by the time I was off the phone with my husband, my torso was impeccably clean and Band-Aid covered,
and Dr. Berson informed me that now we would wait for the
results.

After the biopsy, Dr. Berson graciously gave me one of his
navy-blue scrubs, his name embroidered on the top left corner. Something about the shirt made me feel safe. I folded up
my faux-silk maternity blouse, thankful for it remaining crisp
white, and changed into the scrubs. I exited the biopsy room,
and seeing Dr. Berson in the brightly lit hallway, I started to cry.
It was as if I had stepped out into the unobscured reality of my
circumstances; I could see it now, clearly, right in front of me.

My pregnancies and postpartum months had been my only

experience with having sizeable breasts, and after all my adolescence longing for bigger ones, these boobs were suddenly not all they were cracked up to be. I felt the anger gathering force in my body, rushing up to my throat until I almost yelled at Dr. Berson about my breasts, "I want to get rid of them. Take them. Just take them! I've never had them anyway." Then, finding my breath, I asked him, through tears, "Am I overreacting? I'm pregnant, hormonal, and getting scared. Should I be scared?" Dr. Berson looked at me, sympathetically, and remained silent. I asked him, "What about my husband? I respect his job—we give each other professional freedoms and I don't want to ask him to come home from work after just getting to Phoenix for the week."

"Sometimes family matters come first," he offered. "If I tell you tomorrow that you have breast cancer, would you want him here?"

"Yes."

"Tell him to fly home."

The rest of the daylight hours are difficult to remember. My nervous system, in response to the threat of being in danger, had already started to blur the accumulating moments of that Monday. But I do recall that at the end of the day I thought to myself, *Now is the time a person is supposed to go to bed.* I perfunctorily sat down on my mattress and then assumed the pregnant, side-lying position, a pillow between my bent-knees for support. It was getting late, past 11:00 P.M., but, not surprisingly, I couldn't sleep. I saw that my friend Lee had just posted something onto Facebook; so he's awake, I thought. I messaged him and we were on the phone a few moments later. It felt good to hear his voice and share the fear at my potential news.

I lay in bed, half-awake, half-asleep, waiting for Derek to get home at midnight. He never left the Phoenix airport; he'd got right back onto a return flight to New York City without my ever asking. Lying in the dark, I eventually heard the faint, satisfying click-release of the lock as our apartment door made way for Derek. He silently entered our bedroom, and my eyes caught just the shadow of his beautiful, familiar body—his tall, slender frame, his broad shoulders, the curve of his upper back. His dark gray figure traveled across the room, and then he settled into bed next to me. Bodies close, we held on tight to each other's hands while we slept, not letting go until morning.

What do you do the day you're waiting to find out if you have cancer? The results from the biopsy would come in anytime within the next twenty-four hours. The night before, my friend Lee counseled me to plan fun activities for the day. I told Derek what I really wanted to do was eat a grilled cheese (I was very pregnant!). So down we went to join the others on the city streets. I imagine there must have been joggers and people on their lunch break whizzing by us, going about life as usual, on that perfectly sunny September day, but my vision was narrowed to just me and Derek. Slowly, we walked down Lexington Avenue, our torsos touching, hands clasped together. We were physically attached to one another, like two squares of a sewn quilt. When we arrived at our local diner, on East Seventy-Fifth Street, we sat down at the wooden square table, placed our orders, and my sandwich soon arrived in its melted cheesy glory. As I was about to take a bite, my phone rang. It was Dr. Berson. He said, simply, "It's malignant. Come to my office at four P.M."

2

THE BINDER

Surgical pathology report, dated September 19, 2017

Right breast 1:00 mass, core biopsy:

-Invasive moderately differentiated ductal carcinoma, spanning 13mm in this material, with crush artifact.

Right breast, 11:00 calcification, core biopsy:

-Ductal carcinoma in situ (DCIS), high nuclear grade, solid and cribriform types, with necrosis and calcification.

-Lactational changes.

Lymph node, right axilla, core biopsy:

-Metastatic ductal carcinoma, similar to part A.

The four of us—me, Derek, my mom and dad—sat with Dr. Berson in his office. All I could see was Dr. Berson, the dimmed lights casting a soft glow on his solemn, angular face as he looked at each of us in turn, explaining the results of the biopsy. He warned me to not jump to the conclusion that my cancer was metastatic (which means it had spread throughout my body) just because they found cancer in the lymph nodes. He suggested that I put together a binder with all of my medical information, bring it with me to each appointment, and take notes. "I can do that," I said.

Dr. Berson had already spoken to my three OBGYNs and had set up an appointment with a breast cancer surgeon in New York City whom I would meet with the next day. He assured me that the cancer would not hurt my unborn baby. I told him, through tears, that there was no one else I could have asked for to give me this diagnosis, that he made the most difficult news somehow more bearable through his compassion.

That evening I went by myself to Staples and browsed the folder aisle, looking for just the right binder to house the chaos of imaging slides and Latin-riddled medical reports. It was a familiar setting. I had visited that store many times as a graduate student, seeking index cards and other study aids to help embed novel psychology data to memory. Some of my Rutgers classmates were able to read a text once and the information was then imprinted, permanently, in their minds (this was both amazing and infuriating from my perspective). My brain was less cooperative, and over the many years of being a student I had discovered that I needed to interact with learning material. My go-to study routine involved filling out hundreds of flash cards with my teeny-tiny handwriting, the black words eating up every bit of white space. I remembered it seeming impossible, the notion that I could recruit such a preposterous number of facts to live in my brain. But the act of writing and organizing engendered a sense of agency over my not-knowing. And those Staples purchases—the highlighters, Post-its, extra-fine-tipped pens, index cards, and labels—helped the facts stick and smoothed out my frayed nerves.

I knew how to put things in order, and I desperately needed that skill set to serve me now. This binder search was a task that I could consciously embark upon in an effort to feel in control during what was likely to become an out-of-control situation. Though I recognized, standing in that Staples aisle, that I was no longer the previous version of myself—the doctor-in-training, doing my best to learn and provide effective treatment for my patients. Now *I* was the patient.

The next morning, I felt myself steel over, become soldier-like, shoulders back and head held high, ready for the toils ahead. I was thinking super-rationally, focused on the next steps, the next doctor appointment, what had to be done. I would rise to the challenge. I would give birth to a healthy baby. I would stick around to raise my newborn and my daughter, Sophie. I was in full-on fight mode. This was no time to fall apart.

At the breast surgeon appointment that day, I sat on the examination table covered in semiopaque paper, clothed in another medical gown that managed to wrap around my pregnant belly. I anticipated the moment that the expert, all-knowing doctor would swing open that closed door and translate the foreign land that had become my body. I didn't know it at the time, but this act of waiting—in examination rooms, in doctors' offices, in aptly named waiting rooms—would fill much of my wakeful hours in the weeks and months to come.

The breast surgeon entered the examination room, jet-black-haired, slight in height, and built like a triathlete. She exuded the confidence of a player you would want on your team. My

cancer doctors, thus far, appeared to be Olympians both physically and cognitively. After the breast exam, the surgeon sat
close to me, holding my hands, and in her light blue eyes she
had tears that matched mine. She told me, my husband, and my
parents that she was waiting to receive results of the type of
breast cancer I had, and that would dictate the treatment plan.
However, we would need a PET/CT scan (which takes detailed pictures of the whole body and measures abnormal cell
activity) scheduled for right after my delivery in order to determine whether the cancer had spread beyond the lymph nodes. I
could not officially be assigned a cancer stage without the PET/
CT scan, though a nurse had suggested that I likely had Stage
II breast cancer.

The breast cancer stage model is complex. Challenging my
bias that a bigger number is a better number, in the world of
cancer, the highest number is not the goal. It starts at Stage 0,
which does not translate to zero cancer; it means abnormal cells
are present but considered "precancer" cells. In Stage I, there
is typically the presence of a small tumor. Stage II is generally
marked by a medium-size tumor and the possibility of limited
nearby lymph node involvement. In Stage III, there is often a
larger tumor and "localized spread" to nearby lymph nodes.
Stage IV is characterized by the cancer's "distant spread" beyond the original tissue and lymph nodes to distal parts of the
body.

During our meeting with the breast surgeon after the examination, the mood in her sunlight-filled office was somber. For
the first time in my life, my late grandmother's soothing phrase
everything will be just fine, dearie had met its match. Things were
maybe not going to be just fine. One of the medical interns, sitting in the corner of the office, cried with me, and later, when

it was just the two of us alone, she confided that she, too, had breast cancer years ago. The emotional presence of the surgeon and her staff made me feel like more than a walking diagnosis; they saw me as a mother, a wife, a daughter, a woman who desperately wanted to keep herself and her unborn baby safe. Despite my fear, I was able to recognize their warmth and empathy as a strangely beautiful moment of intimate connection with near strangers.

Midway through the meeting, there was a knock on the door, and pieces of paper were handed to the surgeon. She looked up from the report, smiling, and said that the test indicated that I had Her2 positive breast cancer. She explained that Her2 positive breast cancer patients have too much of a protein called human epidermal growth receptor 2 (Her2), which promotes the growth of cancer cells. Although twenty years ago a Her2 positive diagnosis would have meant a swift death sentence, scientists have since developed effective treatments to target it. The breast surgeon described cure rates as "excellent." So it was very good news that I was Her2 positive! The room breathed a collective sigh of relief.

The meeting with the surgeon was followed by a session with the genetic counselor, then the nurse practitioner, and finally the oncologist. Derek and I took feverish notes, trying to keep up with this new language of chemotherapy agents, immunotherapies, and the schedule of infusions. Twenty weeks of chemo, followed by either a double or single mastectomy (determined by genetic testing), followed by radiation, and immunotherapy infusions for one year. Potential side effects. Where to purchase wigs. To anticipate that my nails may crack or fall off.

All information went dutifully into my accordion binder,

which allowed me to compartmentalize my disease into something manageable, familiar even. By pulling down its cover and securing the elastic band around its case, I was no longer confronted with the impressive array of papers and imaging CDs. All was safely housed in that binder. And I could distance myself from the information it contained.

3

HANNAH

After meeting with the oncologist, I was accompanied upstairs for a tour of the hospital's cancer treatment center. I hoped that I would like it, if possible, although can you ever *like* a chemotherapy infusion area? I remember first noticing the windows, which were covered in a cloudy film and filtered the sunlight into a surreal haze. Older women, I imagine in their sixties or so, sat in the small, characterless waiting room that needed a fresh coat of paint. I was hyperaware of my relatively young age and being nearly nine months pregnant. I did not fit in with this crowd. One of the patients was at the front desk, complaining that she had been waiting too long for her treatment to begin. I looked around and thought, Well, this is pretty depressing.

I peeked into the infusion area. It looked very medical, similar to an emergency room, lacking any of the comforts that would encourage someone to stay put for a while. The chairs appeared stiff, the walls bare, the colors a muted, aseptic grayish-blue. The perimeter of the rectangular treatment suite was divided by hospital privacy curtains, and in each of those closet-size spaces there was a patient hooked up to an IV drip.

Across the suite I saw a tall woman—she was probably in her midforties, with a fedora hat perched upon her almost-bald head with an intentional, slight tilt to the rim. This was a woman who looked as if she were at the ready to socialize at an art gallery or some other cultural event, to schmooze with other well-clad bohemians. Was she famous? She looked like a celebrity and had that dazzle some people just have. She caught my gaze with her gorgeous light-colored eyes, surprising me by breaking the well-known New York City norm that you avert eye contact with strangers, or it must be fleeting at most. On top of that, she smiled—a big, full-mouth smile.

Her, I thought. I want to be like her. She will be my cancer-patient inspiration.

Our stare was interrupted when a nurse led me to a side room for a blood draw, which would be used for my genetic testing. To my relief, the lab technician, a woman with bright blue hair, effortlessly found my historically finicky veins. I started to warm up to the environment; I appreciated that my phlebotomist was permitted, maybe even encouraged, to have fun breaking the "rules" of professional appearance. It was refreshing and comforting, and added levity to the sterile chemotherapy area.

Afterward, back in the waiting room, I asked my guide about the woman in the fedora hat. "Oh, she has a party every time she's here. She has the most rowdy chemo treatments!" Just then the woman emerged from the infusion area, confident and beaming. I approached her and told her, "You are beautiful." She replied in her self-assured voice, "You are beautiful!" and looked at me and my two seemingly cancer-incongruent physical features: my long blond hair and huge pregnant belly. "I dress up for chemo days. I do my makeup and pick out a great outfit. It helps me get through the treatment that way. I'm Hannah,"* she said warmly, still wearing her genuine smile. After I introduced myself, we said our goodbyes and I wished her well—a phrase I had used many times before but hadn't felt the weight of until I shared it with Hannah. There was no exchange of contact information and we never saw each other again.

Can you love someone you've barely met? I hold my memory of Hannah close to me, her smile forever imprinted in my mind. I will be strong like Hannah. I will exude positivity like Hannah. Further along into cancer treatment and presumably out of crisis, Hannah was the living, breathing, and breathtaking evidence that maybe everything was going to be just fine. I could visualize what my future could hold, beyond the immediacy of the present, and I saw that it could look like grace.

Thank you, Hannah.

---

* Name has been changed to protect patient confidentiality.

4

DECISION TIME:
WHEN TO HAVE MY BABY

After deciding upon a cancer treatment plan within just three days of my initial sonogram with Dr. Berson, the next big question was when to give birth. I would be induced, but it was unclear whether to have my baby immediately or wait one more week to get closer to thirty-six weeks. The difference of a few days may seem slight, but if I delivered early, my baby would be more likely to end up in the NICU, lungs not yet fully developed, whereas waiting would mean the baby would likely be born healthy. My various doctors all agreed that I should start chemo within a week or so after delivery, but my treatment team was not initially united about when I should be induced. My breast surgeon was eager for me to give birth sooner rather than later. My OBGYNs were less convinced that I should give birth right away and were trying to figure out the right timetable to balance my health and that of my soon-to-be-born baby.

Sitting around my parents' kitchen table in the apartment I grew up in, my mom, dad, Derek, and I talked through this dilemma. That familiar spot—still adorned with the same fish paintings on the wall, the textured crimson upholstered cushions, my parents' kind eyes resting upon me—flooded me with memories that took place in that very dining nook over the thirty-six years of my life. One time, as kids, my older brother and I pounded packets of Chinese food takeout soy sauce with our fists to see what would happen. To our delight, the brown liquid splattered all over the kitchen wall. Our parents were none too pleased with our "experiment" when they returned from their outing. Slinking my small-framed body underneath the window-nook table when I was finished with a meal, so as not to inconvenience others with having to stand up to let me out (and besides, crawling under furniture is fun). Family meals, the four of us: discussing our days; what we learned at school; early love; and other middle school and then high school theatrics.

But this was a very different problem to solve, and the naivete of my childhood and years as a young adult suddenly felt as if they had shrunken and traveled to a faraway place, like a single water droplet landing at the bottom of a dark, deep well. I was now starting a new kind of life. The precancer days were forever gone.

My father cried as we discussed the options, as he spoke of his love for me and his grandchild. It pained me that my parents were now faced with the reality of having a seriously ill daughter. It wasn't fair; they had already put in their time as devoted caretakers. It was my turn to care for them.

Derek and I were both leaning toward waiting as long as I could before inducing, not only for the physical health of our baby, but also because we could anticipate the significant stress of adding a premature, NICU infant to our already stress-laden lives. The psychological burden of having a baby likely born with health concerns, in addition to my cancer diagnosis, seemed too overwhelming to bear.

Upon being thrust into the world of cancer, I was required to make decisions, and very significant ones, despite being in a state of both shock and fear. Should I consult with more doctors? Why are doctors recommending different chemotherapy regimens? Whose treatment plan sounds the best? Who do I feel most comfortable with interpersonally? Do I follow my OBGYN's, oncologist's, or surgeon's advice about when to give birth? When do *I* want to give birth?

I was determined to stay clearheaded, to make the best decisions I could, given the information available, and as quickly as possible. My sympathetic nervous system, and more specifically, the "fight" of the fight-flight stress response, had been galvanized. Since the threat of cancer was an abstract concept that required considerable problem-solving, expedient decisiveness was my version of being a wild animal fighting for its survival.

The decision was made. Together, my family and medical team agreed to schedule my induction for exactly thirty-six weeks, when our baby would be more likely to arrive healthy.

TIME TO TELL SOPHIE

On a summer evening in Tucson in 2006, Tom Boyle witnessed a teenager being hit by a car and then dragged underneath it for twenty feet down the street.[1] Boyle immediately ran toward the car, and in a surge of superhero-like strength was able to lift the car off of the boy. How was Boyle able to achieve that impossible feat? The body is capable of engaging in extraordinary actions during the fight-or-flight surge of nervous system excitement.[2] In moments of significant threat, we are flooded with adrenaline, triggering a "jolt" of energy and vigilance.[3] Our heart and breathing rates increase, and blood supply is directed to our muscles, allowing them to contract with greater force.[4] At the same time, our perception of pain is dulled with the brain's release of opioids and endocannabinoids.[5] In fact, as Boyle made his way home after saving that teenager's life, he realized that he had clenched his jaw so hard while lifting the car that he had shattered eight of his teeth. The pain signals that typically would have alerted him to put down that heavy weight had been temporarily quieted.

Though Sophie was not physically in danger, I knew that psychologically, she was in harm's way. Yet despite my physical frailty, the stress of the cancer diagnosis had aroused an extreme, and adaptive, fight response. I felt a highly effective mode of functioning take over my body, a summoning of energy, focus, and strength that I never knew I had. It was my version of lifting a thousand-pound car.

Derek and I knew that a difficult conversation would need to take place with Sophie. But how do you tell your four-year-old child that you have cancer? She didn't know what that word meant, and actually, that not-knowing was likely a blessing. I knew, however, that she was about to see her mommy not only feeling very sick, looking dramatically different, with no hair, eyebrows, or eyelashes, but also be unable to play with her as I had in the past. And these changes would be both scary and frustrating for her.

We sought out advice about how to best convey my diagnosis to Sophie: the social worker at the cancer center; my therapist; and Sophie's preschool directors. After painstaking thought and attention to specific language (do we use the C word?), we devised a plan. And one morning, we joined Sophie on the floor as she was playing and told her that we needed to talk with her about something.

She looked at us, quietly, intensely, as if she sensed the seriousness of the conversation. Derek said, "Mama is sick and will be in bed more than usual. She has something called 'cancer,' and it's different from the colds we usually get. You can't get the cancer from her—it's not catchy like when we have a runny nose."

I added, "It will take a while for me to get better but I will get better." I paused, and then asked, "Do you have any questions?" She shook her head, no. Sophie then turned her small body away from us, silently. With her back to us, she made fists, hit the floor with them, and then went back to playing.

This conversation would be the first in a series of "updates" we gave Sophie throughout my treatment, as we were advised to provide brief and factual information about the very near future as it became relevant. For example, we were instructed *not* to tell Sophie that I was going to lose my hair until right before my hair fell out. At each new stage, she could prepare for the shifts in my appearance and functioning. The emphasis was on how my illness would impact her and my relationship with her.

At the hospital just days after my initial appointment with Dr. Berson, I had signed a consent form to begin treatment, and the goal written out by the nurse read: CURE. All signs pointed to a challenging year ahead, no doubt, but my medical team appeared confident that I would survive and become cancer-free. Death was never part of the conversation. So there was nothing to be gained from sharing with Sophie that, sometimes, cancer takes away life.

Her first and only experience with death had taken place just a year prior, when she was three years old. We were in the country, on a lawn, when she found a tiny green bug, probably a mini-grasshopper, on her leg. Scared, she asked me to get the bug off of her. I said, "Oh, that's just a 'sweetie pie'! Look, they're nice. Nothing to be scared of." I placed the bug on my arm and quickly found more in the grass, adding them to my hand. Soon enough, Sophie wanted to do the same, and was collecting her sweetie pies to let them crawl on her hand and arm. She started singing to them, as if they were her babies she was trying to calm with a lullaby.

Then there was a shriek. Sophie had picked up another sweetie pie between her thumb and forefinger, and had mistakenly used too much force. She had unintentionally crushed the bug, and saw it smashed, motionless, between her fingers. She began to cry hysterically, her face stricken and tears streaming down her cheeks. I consoled her and she eventually went back to playing with her new bug friends, albeit more gently.

Sophie had learned that there can be life, and then there can not be life. Did she understand, in that moment, the permanence of death?

I was not ready to explain that concept to her.

HAIR

"I would cut your hair before you begin treatment, so that you, and Sophie, can adjust to your new look," said Mimi, the preschool director. In addition to providing our family with enormous practical and emotional support, the staff members of Sophie's preschool were always at the ready to share thoughtful parenting suggestions about how to navigate my illness. And so, following teacher's orders, I booked a haircut for later that week.

At the hospital, the oncology nurse told me that the two chemotherapy agents I was slated to begin shortly "result in total hair loss." With her brown eyes looking straight into mine she warned, "It can be psychologically traumatizing to lose your hair." I was struck by her use of the words "psychologically traumatizing," a phrase I had uttered so often to my own patients to normalize our reactions to abnormal experiences—but now it was my turn to prepare myself for a cancer-induced emotional assault. She urged me to consider "cold capping," which can reduce hair loss for many women. Before, during, and after the chemotherapy infusion, a hired cold cap professional would place freezing (–22 degrees Fahrenheit) helmet-like hats on my head, alternating them every twenty minutes or so to maintain the frigid temperatures on my scalp. Similar to cold packs that people use to reduce back, knee, or other body pains, these blue, gel-filled scalp caps would be secured in place with Velcro straps. I was told that cold capping is uncomfortable; not surprisingly, it causes headaches similar to a "brain freeze" sensation, makes your whole body feel cold, and would lengthen my infusion day by many hours.

With Sophie at home and a baby on the way, I barely considered cold capping as an option. Adding time at the hospital for a 10 to 100 percent chance (quite an uncertain range) of saving only a portion of my hair was not compelling.[1] And, I *despise* being cold. When I was a baby, my mom endured my wails whenever she pushed me in my stroller during the winter months in New York City. An attempt at a family ski trip when I was five years old resulted in me refusing to go outside except to have my picture taken in full gear, posing in the snow as if I were a professional skier, then back inside to the kids' care room with my coloring books. Strapping freezing cold caps around my head would have derailed my goal to make the infusions as stress-free and comfortable as possible.

So I had resigned myself to the notion that I would go bald. As a teenager, I had felt the occasional urge to buzz my hair but was never brave enough to go through with it. In a way, I saw this as my opportunity to finally get a version of the Irish singer Sinéad O'Connor's look that I had admired years ago. Her appearance (and voice) were equal parts pure beauty and rebellion, which I yearned for myself as a fourteen-year-old. I had settled on nonconforming outfits like an unbuttoned Salvation Army extra-large pajama shirt with a psychedelic 1970s crop top beneath, vintage bell-bottom jeans, and combat boots. I pierced a line of holes in my ears, in my belly button, and ultimately, my nose. But I always felt that I had wimped out a bit by holding on to my tresses.

I had actually gone the opposite route from Sinéad for over twenty years. My thick blond hair cascaded in waves down to the small of my back. It was so long that I was able to wrap my hair around itself to form a bun, self-contained, atop my head. My husband would refer to my hair as my mane. I had tried to tame it in high school, spending twenty minutes every morning blow-drying it stick straight. And then I calculated how much time I had spent straightening my hair (121 hours per year) and decided to try to embrace its wildness. Thereafter, it became my primary physical feature.

When the time came to cut my hair, my mom insisted on taking me to her hairstylist, whom she had contacted prior to the appointment to prepare him for what would likely be an emotional shear. When we arrived at the fancy salon, I learned that since my hair was not dyed, I could donate it. I had briefly considered getting a wig made from my own hair, but the $5,000 price tag scrapped that idea. My hair would become a wig, but it would sit upon another cancer patient's head. I brought photographs of inspiration for the hairstylist but emphasized that the look of choice was Mia Farrow circa *Rosemary's Baby*. I recognized that I was asking for her hairstyle with my belly protruding with a baby, too, and joked that I'd take the pixie cut without the devil baby, please. Though there was also something foreign, sinister, and dangerous growing in my body.

The stylist misted my hair and combed it into sections, tying each one off with an elastic band one-inch from my scalp. By the end of this process, I resembled a blond version of Medusa with ten damp ponytails sprouting from my head. One by one, the ponies were snipped right above the elastic band, and the long tendrils were placed in my and my mother's laps. Then an assistant came over and collected the ponies, placed them in a see-through plastic bag, and took them away.

The other women at the hair salon quickly figured out what was happening with this pregnant girl, tears in her eyes, cutting off all of her long hair while clutching her mother's hand. Seeing my vastly different reflection in the mirror filled me with a sense of loss for my previous healthy, long-haired self. But then I caught the salon women's eyes on me; I was surrounded by support and felt a surge of empowerment. The new do made me feel a bit tougher, like I had added another weapon to my armory to fight this fight. I had cut my hair off before the toxic chemotherapy agents would have their way with it. I thought to myself, Cancer, you just lost this battle—I took my hair before you could.

Later that day, waiting for my next doctor's appointment, I looked down at my wrist. There was a black hair band wrapped around it, ready for when I often needed to pull my hair back into a quick bun or braid. I stared and realized—I have had a black hair tie around my wrist for as long as I can remember. There has just always been one there, like a tattooed bracelet. I had no use for it now. What would my wrist feel like without it? As I removed the hair tie, I found a long strand of my blond hair twisted around the band. My stomach flipped.

The last strand of my hair—the final remnant of my pre-cancer appearance. I thought, What do I do with it? Should I honor it somehow? Simply throw it out? I played with the hair between my fingers, felt its texture, examined its length, its curvature, its shape. I said goodbye to that strand of pale, glistening yellow, and then stood up from the waiting room chair and threw it in the garbage.

7

BIRTHDAY

My induction was scheduled for a Monday evening so that my baby would be born the next morning, at exactly thirty-six weeks gestation. It was a busy day. Derek was at the closing for our first purchased home, another significant life-changing event. I was packing my hospital bag and finalizing the décor in the nursery for our newborn.

When Derek and I arrived at the hospital we were taken to a birthing room where I was told that I would begin a Pitocin (induction medication) drip shortly. Although I had hoped to try for a drug-free birth when I delivered Sophie, I ended up getting induced. As this second birth was now a planned induction, my OB and I had agreed that I would receive an epidural.

So Derek and I were surprised and disappointed (I had actually been looking forward to the numbness, since my right hip area had been in pain for so many months that the idea of not feeling the lower part of my body sounded like bliss) when our OB told us that the anesthesiologist had refused to administer the epidural. The doctor, aware of my breast cancer diagnosis, was concerned that the cancer could have potentially spread to my back. She informed us that if an epidural were injected into cancer cells, there would be risk of permanent paralysis. The anesthesiology team insisted that I get an MRI to check my back for any tumors before proceeding with the epidural. The induction was on hold.

Squeezed into the dark cylinder of the MRI machine, I felt the pressure of contractions, most likely stress-induced. I focused on my breathing, trying to calm down my overwhelmed mind and body, despite the cacophony of the jackhammer-like electronic sounds. Back in the birthing room, I was told that the results of the MRI looked good, but the head anesthesiologist wanted another MRI just to be sure. Into the machine I went, for the second time. This time, the contractions intensified. I tried to stay still, but at times was writhing in labor pain, trapped in that deafening, white cage-like tube.

I was relieved to be out of the machine and back in my dimly lit, quiet, relatively spacious (as compared to an MRI, most places are) birthing room. Then my OB walked into the delivery room with a strange look on her face. She told me and Derek, calmly, but with what seemed like disbelief, that the head anesthesiologist believed that he saw cancer "lesions" in my back. Though the test was inconclusive, it meant that I would not be eligible for an epidural.

I think my OB sat down next to me. I think she may have touched my arm—she made some gesture of being human with another suffering human, of caring deeply.

What I do remember was how Derek and I sat on the hospital bed, holding each other's bodies up despite the feeling of collapse, of air being ripped from our lungs. The room, too, felt as if it had been sucked dry of its oxygen. Yet I summoned the breath to cry into him. The mind-bending reality was that I had just been told that I may have metastatic breast cancer. This was a terminal disease, and the goal of CURE from my earlier records evaporated. In a few hours, I would give birth to a helpless infant, whom I maybe would never get to know. Who would never get to know me. I called out, "Am I going to live to take care of my baby? Who's going to take care of my babies?!?"

No one could answer me.

I had to put those thoughts aside because, for now, my focus needed to be on my baby being born safely. I held on to the word "inconclusive" and to the first MRI, which had "looked good." I had also been moving during the MRIs because of contractions. So maybe—I hoped—the imaging was unclear and misleading? A PET/CT scan later that week would yield the actual results.

The delivery options were as follows: (1) start the induction and deliver without an epidural, or (2) C-section under general anesthesia. With Sophie, my body had been strong. I had trained it for labor with prenatal yoga classes and cardiovascular exercises. This time around, my body was weak, my muscles atrophied from disuse. The hip pain, barely manageable when *not* in labor, seemed like it would be unbearable if I actually needed to push a baby out of my body, past those bones and ligaments that constantly felt like they were on fire. I couldn't imagine mustering the energy, physical or mental, to labor and deliver a baby without adequate pain management. I decided to get the C-section, and the wait for the operating room began.

Lying on the operating table just prior to being knocked out by anesthesia, I asked my OBs (two from the group practice were there to perform the C-section) if they could "take a look" at my organs when they opened me up to see if there were any tumors. They assured me that they would. And off I went, into the ether. Minutes later, I became a mother to a second baby girl.

Siena was born healthy. The C-section was a success with no complications. My OBs also reported that they had "looked around" and hadn't seen any tumors. I imagined them rummaging around my insides, as if searching in a drawer for a pair of socks. It was a relief to hear that they hadn't opened me up to find my insides teeming with cancerous lesions. That was enough reassurance for me to focus on what was most important in that moment: my child.

At the maternity ward I was led to a small private room at the quiet end of the hallway that the hospital staff, in their great empathy, had gifted me. It was in this room that Derek and I would get to know our cuddly, beautiful, miraculous daughter. I wondered, How could she be so perfect after growing inside my cancerous body? Siena would be my last child, as I was told that chemotherapy would shut down my ovaries and put me into early menopause. She had been created and developed just in the nick of time. I was so lucky to have her.

That room on the maternity ward became its own universe, in another galaxy away from where my cancer diagnosis existed. Derek and I hardly made mention of it. It was almost like an unspoken rule. He had asked family members to not bring up my diagnosis during the maternity stay, so that I could have the opportunity to be fully present in the moment to bond with my baby. The focus was solely on Siena, on welcoming her to the world, on getting to know each other and introducing her to her big sister, Sophie. Those four days were spent with us two parents being dopey in love, snuggling up to our little newborn.

After the first day of initial C-section pain, I started to walk and noticed that my hip pain was gone. Totally, completely gone. Physical therapists and doctors throughout my pregnancy had told me that my baby's head was positioned into my right hip area, and that was the cause of the pain. Now that Siena had been born, the pain had lifted. I was euphoric when I shared the news with Derek; the implication was that perhaps there was no cancer spread beyond my breast and lymph nodes. My body had been in pain simply because carrying around a weighty baby can be tough on joints.

A day or so later, the hip pain returned. The anesthesia had worn off.

8

LEOPARD

PET/CT scan findings, dated October 9, 2017

CHEST: Physiologic FDG avidity is seen in mediastinal blood pool, myocardium. Multiple FDG avid foci right breast, SUV up to 7.9

THORACIC NODES: Multiple FDG avid right subpectoral/axillary nodes, SUV up to 4.6

HEPATOBILIARY: FDG avid focus, SUV 7.9 left liver lobe. Liver background SUV mean, as a reference for comparing FDG, is 2.0

BONES/SOFT TISSUES: FDG avid foci anterior abdominal wall, probably postsurgical inflammatory changes. A more nodular appearing FDG avid focus anterior abdominal wall, sequence 3, image 183, possibly postsurgical inflammatory. Multiple widespread FDG avid lytic lesions of the axial and appendicular skeleton, for example T1 vertebra SUV 11.2; sternum SUV 10.1; L1 vertebra SUV 9.0; sacrum SUV 11.3; right ischial bone SUV 12.1. Lytic bone metastases demonstrate partly soft tissue components, for example right lateral seventh rib. Fracture right posterior 11th rib. Extensive lytic lesions right pubic/ischial bone and right acetabulum seen with probably fracture in the region of the right ischium. In the region of the spine osseous lytic lesions involve partly posterior vertebral cortex, for example C2 vertebra, L3 vertebra.

You can't eat or drink for six hours before a PET/ CT scan. One week after Siena's birth, I arrived at the testing center with an empty belly and was given a large jug of magenta-hued liquid to drink, a glucose concoction that, once in my system, would light up areas of my body in which the cancer was active. Apparently, cancer, like us humans, is a fan of sweets. I was also injected with a radioactive isotope. The blue-robed medical professional carefully removed the tiny syringe of fluid from a metal canister kept inside a larger refrigerated metal canister. There was a dramatic *tssssssss* sound upon opening each container. And then into my vein it went. I was told to stay away from my daughters for the next twelve to twenty-four hours since I would be radioactive from the injection. I imagined my body haloed in an orange, pulsating light invisible to the human eye.

The results from the PET/CT scan were going to get back to me later that day, in time for the appointment with my oncologist. It was then that I would officially learn what stage cancer I had, if it had spread beyond the lymph nodes, and if so, where.

My family and I sat in the examining room, waiting for Dr. Dang's arrival. My brother had flown into the city for the appointment, all the way across the United States from his home in Idaho. We arranged the chairs in the room and sat in a line— Derek, me, my brother, my dad, my mom.

Dr. Dang opened the door. I searched her face for any hints about the results, but she was expressionless, perhaps a practiced stoicism. She sat down in front of me and looked me straight in the eyes and said, "Are you ready?" I knew then that the news was not good. I nodded yes, meeting her gaze.

With the utmost sensitivity and care, Dr. Dang said that the cancer had been found in my breast and lymph nodes, as we already knew. But it was also in my bones and in my liver.

My liver? I was dumbfounded. Dr. Dang continued to speak, but her sentences floated away, and the only word I could grasp on to was *liver*. It had never occurred to me that my liver would be at risk of disease. I kept saying out loud in disbelief, "My liver?! My liver?!"

It was now official: I had been diagnosed with Stage IV, metastatic breast cancer. Confused, I looked at my family members' faces for some understanding. Did you just hear her say that, too? Everyone had an identical expression—wide-eyed fear. Derek tells me that he had been sobbing at the news. For me, I remember no sound in the room. Time felt as if it had stopped, my sensory system on shutdown. That moment started to feel like a movie, and I was somehow an actor playing the part of a cancer patient. In psychology-speak, we call this phenomenon *dissociation*. In times of great stress, we can feel removed from our bodies, as if we're watching our lives unfold from outside of our selves.

Urgent words spewed out of my mouth toward Dr. Dang, "What does this mean?!?" and "How much longer do I have to live?!?" She replied, with clear empathy, "Years." I noted the vagueness of her answer and pushed for greater clarity. She didn't budge but did offer, "I have women with your diagnosis who have been with me for twenty years." I didn't ask about the other women.

Later when I looked at the PET/CT scan image, I saw that I

had become a leopard, spotted with cancer from neck to thigh. The light gray "normal" of the scan was taken over almost completely by dark gray splotches in my breast, liver, and, most densely, throughout my bones. I had a fracture in one of my ribs, a sign that the cancer had weakened my skeleton to the point of breakage.

Dr. Dang informed us of the new treatment plan. Since the cancer had spread beyond the breast and throughout my body, there was no way to effectively remove it with surgery or radiation. So those modes of intervention were now off the table. We would start immunotherapy (Herceptin and Perjeta) immediately. Chemotherapy (Taxol) as soon as my C-section had healed. An injection called Xgeva to build a bone-like substance where the cancer had eaten away at my bones. I would receive chemotherapy for six months and immunotherapy infusions for the rest of my life. The revised goal would be to "TREAT" the cancer. That initial plan to "CURE" it had vanished, as did the hope of survival.

Dr. Dang also made mention that we would start with the plan above, and if/when it stopped working, we would have other treatments to explore. So from the outset, there was an expectation that the chemotherapy and immunotherapies might not hold my cancer at bay.

Dr. Dang left the room, saying that she would give us a moment to be alone as a family. The five of us stood up, formed a tight circular hug with me at its center, and cried together.

In my conversations with other cancer patients since my diagnosis, I have noted that many of us (we are an "us") get stuck on a certain thought. And we ruminate, obsess, chew, and chew some more on this thought, which truly serves no valid purpose. I'd worked with many patients in my psychology practice to help them disengage from this cognitive process but found myself unable to detach from one particularly stubborn thought after that telling visit: How much time do I have left? And all the thoughts that spun out from there: How long will my girls have their mother? Will I see Sophie grow up and discover the world around her? Will we continue our nightly ritual of books and snuggles? The recapping of her day's events, our heads touching while sharing her pillow, her bedroom lit by the soft glow of her star night-light? Will I help Siena take her first steps? Will I get to know her personality, and will she get to know mine? Will I be there for the girls when they need me? A scraped knee, a broken heart?

Despite my fixation on the amount of time I had left to live, I had decided to honor my initial promise to myself to avoid the internet at all costs and to save all questions for my oncologist only (lesson learned from my googling months prior). So, despite my years of searching databases for research articles as a doctoral student, and knowledge that there were likely statistics relevant to my diagnosis, I steered clear. I knew that the stats were going to offer neither comfort nor hope.

Prediagnosis, I had heard and uttered the word "metastatic" before, but at times had unintentionally added an *s* or left out an *a* (mestastic or metastatis), unaware of the proper spelling or pronunciation of the term, let alone its meaning.

"Metastatic," or "advanced," cancer is the most deadly form because when cancer spreads to different areas of the body, it becomes increasingly difficult to treat. Common areas of metastatic breast cancer spread include the bones, liver, lungs, and brain. The more organ systems involved, the worse the prognosis.

Before my official Stage IV diagnosis, I had a sinking suspicion that I had cancer in my bones, though I had no insight into
that suspicion's implications. I was not aware of the huge gulf
that lies between nonmetastatic and metastatic cancer, that one
is curable and the other is not. In my irrational, denial-laden
mind, I had somehow convinced myself that if the cancer were
in my bones, it could be eradicated with proper treatment. In reality, that outcome is rarely the case. I was operating under the
unsophisticated notion that treating a bone with cancer is similar to treating a broken bone—you wear a cast, and the bone
heals. But it's not so simple. In fact, once the cancer spreads
to a distal part of the body, you land squarely in metastatic-
land, with the odds stacked well against your ever returning to
a cancer-free life. My utter bafflement at the discovery of the
disease in my liver (it invaded a vital organ!) was the wake-up
call that finally made me realize, *Oh my God, this will likely kill
me, and soon.*

Just how soon? Setting aside my fear of the hard facts, I dug
up metastatic breast cancer research articles for the first time
approximately eight months after my initial diagnosis. I wasn't
ready, emotionally, to read the grim statistics until then. The
so-called Cleopatra Trial investigated the effects of Herceptin,
Perjeta, and chemotherapy (my treatments) among Her2 positive metastatic breast cancer patients (my diagnosis). In the
article, Her2 positive metastatic breast cancer is described as
"aggressive" and with a "poor prognosis."[1] The Cleopatra
researchers found that the combination of the cancer-fighting
agents above resulted in a "median overall survival [of] 56.5
months."[2] Translation: on average, the women with my diagnosis who received the treatment I was about to begin lived for
four to five years. The findings were "significant" because Per-

jeta, a relatively newer immunotherapy agent, added an average of approximately fifteen months to patients' lives as compared to those who received only Herceptin and chemotherapy. So I would be lucky to be alive at forty-two years old. I would likely be dead before Sophie would be nine and Siena five.

9

I FEEL IT IN MY BONES

As my C-section incision had not fully sealed one week out from the birth, Dr. Dang said that we would hold off on chemotherapy, which can interfere with wound healing. But, she said, we would start immunotherapy immediately and described the treatments (Herceptin and Perjeta) as "potent" agents that could shrink down my rapidly dividing cancer cells.

Derek, my mom, and my brother accompanied me to my first infusion. When we arrived in the treatment room, my brother revealed a large canvas-like bag and began to unpack its contents, handing each item to me, one by one: a Kindle and headphones; lavender oil for relaxation; peppermint oil to fight nausea; a travel blanket to cuddle up in; sucking candies to remove the chemo-induced metallic taste in my mouth; shea butter cream and lip balm to protect my skin from cracking. My brother and sister-in-law had surprised me by creating my chemotherapy coping bag with all things distracting and soothing to use during my treatment days.

Having my older brother with me during the most stressful, scary time in my life provided me with a comfort that is difficult to put into words.

Ben has always made me feel wanted, even when I was a total pain-in-the-ass kid. He accepted my quirks and treated me as an equal despite his being seven years my senior. He put up with my ridiculous protests, like the time when I sat between him and his high school friend Mick in the backseat of my parents' car. The two boys were listening to music together on a CD player with the help of a y-jack wire, which rested weightlessly over my lap. In what felt like an assault to my personal space I yelled, "Owwww! BEN! This wire is *burning* my leg!" In all likelihood, my father intervened with his frequent driving line, "If you don't start behaving, I'm going to turn the car around." That was enough to shut me up.

Somehow, my brother was kind and patient enough to not only tolerate my neuroses but even invite me to spend time with him. During his junior and senior years of high school, he routinely hosted poker night for his friends at our family's apartment. It was a given that I would be seated at that oval mahogany table with all the guys, glaringly out of place as a preteen girl. But it didn't seem to matter. At each new hand, they named the poker game of choice, and would remind me of the rules as necessary. It was a blast. I mean, how many seventeen-year-old brothers do you know who would include their ten-year-old sister at poker night?

Ben is now a surgeon in Idaho with a demanding practice and the father of two incredible kids. For those early days of my treatment, he was by my side constantly. We often didn't need to speak, but I would lean into him, literally, for support.

If we were seated next to each other, my torso would automatically assume a forty-five-degree angle to rest my head upon his shoulder. In our silence there was a deep sense of our mutual affection.

When he wasn't able to be physically present in New York City, he would call into every doctor appointment with my oncologist. On the speakerphone, he asked medical questions that the rest of us never would have known to ask. He was doing his job not only as a doctor, but also as my big brother, trying to protect his little sister.

I've always known that I'm one of the lucky ones, to have such a devoted, kind, and thoughtful family. My parents and brother are good to the core. There are still the inevitable conflicts that arise in any family, but after my diagnosis, those silly irritations all but disappeared from our relationships with one another. What was left was only love, and hoping to be together for as long as we possibly could.

On a Sunday evening, less than a week after I had started immunotherapy, my friends Lauren and Sam visited with me. I was in bed as usual, keeping my movements to a minimum to curb the discomfort in my hip, which was just as bad as it had been when I was pregnant. They cozied up with me in my bedroom, providing support and laughter and the full-hearted feeling that comes from being with people who are like a chosen family to you.

I'm not sure when it hit—the pain so excruciating that I started screaming—but I do remember that I had been trying to get myself out of my bed to go to the bathroom, which was approximately ten feet away. Lauren and Sam were on either side of me, holding me up with all of their strength, trying to help me make it over the several yards to the bathroom. All three of us were crying. I couldn't make it; it was too far, the pain too violent.

Much of that night is not accessible to me. It's probably stored somewhere deep in my memory, in a place where I don't have the language to understand or describe it. I do remember my mother showing up, and along with Derek, their agreeing to call 911. I don't remember being put on the stretcher. Or the trip in the ambulance. But once I was at the cancer urgent care center, I do remember being told that I would need to be admitted to the hospital in order to get the pain under control.

Over those four days at the hospital, a team of doctors devised a plan to reduce my pain. I would wear a fentanyl patch and take morphine pills as needed for breakthrough pain. I underwent additional X-ray and CT scans, which revealed that the bone lesions were:

> *extensive, predominantly lytic osseous metastases in lower lumbar spine, pelvis, and proximal femurs. The largest metastasis is located in medial wall and posterior column of right acetabulum, extending into ischial tuberosity and ischial ramus, with multiple areas of cortical destruction. Lytic metastasis in body of right pubic bone extends throughout inferior pubic ramus, with multiple areas of cortical destruction.*

Pain management via opioids would not be enough to address the "largest metastasis" that had entangled itself throughout my pelvic and hip area. So I began radiation treatment for palliative purposes. In order to prepare for the radiation, I was tattooed with four permanent black ink spots so that the technician could perfectly align a brace-like shield over the areas of my body that were to be protected from the rays. Then the radiation was administered to my right pelvic area twice per day during my hospital stay.

I almost got used to the transferring of my body—which was now merely a long, stiff, rectangular mass—from hospital cot to radiation gurney. The two people on either side of me saying, "Ready? One, two, three, LIFT!" I was immobile and did not know whether I would ever be able to move myself on my own.

Each morning, Derek biked from our apartment, where Siena was now two weeks old, to the hospital to spend the day with me. I have fleeting recollections of his presence, but mostly I just remember pain. I can't imagine what it must have been like for him and my mom to behold me in such a state.

One day at the hospital, I suffered from a severe headache, migraine-like in sharpness and intensity. I squinted my eyes shut, my hands gripped my forehead and temples, and I was unable to speak. The medical team took one look at me and off I went for another CT scan. Derek, my mom, and I anxiously awaited the results, dreading what seemed to be the all-too-possible reality that the cancer had spread to my brain. We all sighed in relief when the results came back clean. There was no evidence of cancer spread to my brain. Not yet, at least. Derek has since shared with me that he feared that I was not going to leave that hospital alive.

I do not remember what we told Sophie about why Mama was away from home for four nights. I do not know if she awoke that Sunday evening to hear my harrowing shrieks of pain. Thankfully, we had round-the-clock help with Sophie and Siena in anticipation of my beginning chemotherapy, so my children were safe and well cared for. But I worried about Sophie and Siena, and how their little minds were trying to make sense of their mommy's screams, and then absence.

When my pain went from searing to a dull ache, I was discharged from the hospital, but with a new accessory. I would have to use a walker at all times. I was a "fall risk," and if I did in fact fall there was a high probability of fracturing my damaged bones. There was no mention of whether this walker would be temporary. The hospital staff wasn't able to tell me if I would ever be able to walk again without it.

Back home I went, into my familiar bed, to a space that had been set up to be my cancer-fighting room. Derek had brought our TV into the bedroom and had compiled a list of my favorite 1980s movies for us to watch together. He also brought in a chair for visitors to sit in. (Though my friends and family members usually opted to hang out on the bed.) I had everything I needed in our bedroom to get me through my treatment days.

Siena was brought to me for snuggles and bottle feedings. In the week after her birth, my breasts swelled with milk; they sat heavy on my chest, ever-present reminders that my body was eager to nourish my infant. But my immunotherapy and morphine-rich milk was not safe for little Siena. I considered placing cabbage leaves on my breasts, as I had heard they reduce milk production. But with all the goings-on, cabbage leaves never materialized in our apartment. Instead, I waited for my body to figure out that I would not be bringing my newborn baby to my breasts, and my milk dried up.

My children were my constant companions. Siena was just the perfect size to hold in my arms without making me strain. She slept on me. Nuzzled into me. And with my Sophie, all of the "screen-time" rules Derek and I had previously enforced were immediately abandoned. Sophie climbed carefully into bed with me to watch movies and kid TV shows. We would read together. We would gently cuddle. My girls filled me up with joy and love and gratitude.

Mostly numbed-out on opioids, and with the walker holding me stable, I was able to slowly move through my small apartment. Anything on the floor or that involved bending was out of the question. Derek helped me dress, put on my socks and shoes. I felt elderly and frail. But I convinced myself that despite my outward appearance, I was strong enough to start the next phase of the cancer fight.

10

THE FIRST DRIP

I can't say that I was excited to start chemo, but I was eager to have the cancer-killing substance coursing through my body. My mom relayed her cancer-survivor friend Elise's helpful visualization: chemotherapy would be like Pac-Man, traveling through the mazelike alleyways of my insides, gobbling up the diseased cells wherever it went. The chemotherapy treatment had already been pushed back two weeks from our initial plan, so I was especially eager for Pac-Man to start his work.

After I got the green light from Dr. Dang that my C-section scar was adequately healed three weeks post C-section, I was off to the infusion room with my walker, Mom, and Derek. I was uneasy about the potential chemo side effects: the nausea, mouth sores, increased susceptibility to infection, neuropathy (tingling and numbness in hands and feet), cracking skin and nails, and baldness. But I was ready to take them on.

My infusion nurse, Ellie, talked us through the Taxol administration procedure and the unlikely possibility of an allergic reaction, which causes flushing (facial reddening) and anaphylaxis.[1] She found my vein with ease, hooked me up to the IV, and the first drop of Taxol was released into the plastic tubing, traveling into my bloodstream.

I felt my throat close. I couldn't breathe. I tried to speak but was only able to force out a tiny, suppressed grunt. Ellie, on alert for an allergic response, said, quietly, "This is it." I felt my face turn as bright and hot as red coals. I silently reached out my arms to Derek and my mom. There was no air reaching my lungs.

Within an instant, Ellie had turned off the Taxol drip, alerted the hospital nursing team, and administered Benadryl into my vein. About six members of the nursing team rushed into the room. One carried an oxygen tank and deftly wrapped a breathing tube around my head and placed the cannula up my nostrils. I still felt like I couldn't breathe, though the staff calmly and empathically explained that I had gotten the necessary medications and would be OK.

Dr. Dang appeared in the treatment room soon after and sat with me. I was still terrified and trying to find my breath, but she assured me that I was now safe. She told me that Taxol would clearly not be my chemotherapy agent, but that there were many others we could use in its stead. My breathing started to regulate, and I was feeling sleepy from the Benadryl. It was decided that I had been through enough for one day, and we could reschedule the chemotherapy for when I felt better.

I shook my head. No. I came to get chemotherapy that day, and I wasn't planning on leaving the center until I had gotten my first full dose. I didn't want to push back chemo yet another week—or longer. Dr. Dang asked me if I was sure. I was.

Without missing a beat, she described the new chemotherapy we would use, called Vinorelbine. It has fewer side effects as

compared with Taxol, though is toxic to veins when injected
and destroys them over time. I would need a port placement (a
central line on my upper chest for direct access to my bloodstream) in order to avoid venous irritation and uncomfortable
arm/hand sensations, which could be temporary or permanent.
But today, we would take on the side effect risks and use my vein
for treatment.

After a few hours, my breathing had returned to normal and
I woke from a Benadryl-induced nap. I was ready for my first
infusion of Vinorelbine. The nurse asked if I felt pain at the
site of the IV, which could indicate that the chemotherapy had
escaped into my surrounding tissue and could cause "significant
damage" (what that meant, I did not know, and did not want to
find out). I told my nurse that I felt no pain. The Vinorelbine
was in my vein, starting its Pac-Man pursuit.

PART II

BETRAYAL

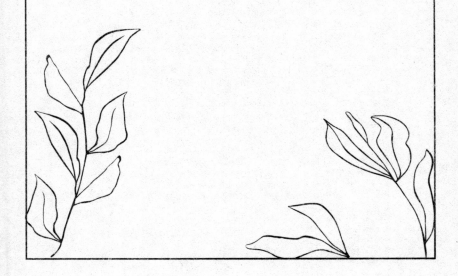

11

ARE YOU MY CANCER?

I am a statistical anomaly. Thirty-six years old (0.44 percent likelihood of developing breast cancer within one's thirties), diagnosed with breast cancer during pregnancy (approximately one out of every three thousand pregnancies), and Stage IV at diagnosis (only 6 to 10 percent of new breast cancer cases).[1, 2, 3] With no risk factors and no genetic loading, it's no wonder that the cancer diagnosis made zero sense to me.

Where the hell did it come from? In my anger and confusion, I searched desperately for an explanation.

There were moments of ostensible discovery. Catching sight of my oral retainer in my medicine cabinet—could that be the culprit? Or what about that antisweating prescription medication that I used as a teenager? Was it exposure to chemicals during my high school senior trip? The hotel had been under major construction, and two other classmates on the trip with me were diagnosed with cancer in their thirties, too. Isn't that too big of a coincidence? Or did I eat too much cured meat? Maybe it was my habit of ordering takeout dinners in BPA-laden plastic containers from New York City restaurants? Is there something in my current daily routine that is silently switching on the cancer cells in my body, allowing them to grow wild?

Almost everything—shampoo, car exhaust, a tuna fish sandwich—was now scrutinized as a possible cancer-causer, and I felt helpless to keep myself safe as the "what ifs" swirled around my head.

Four years later, I still don't know what caused my cancer. In all likelihood, I never will.

Many of my patients struggle with the same psychological conundrum: anxiety in the face of the unknown. Situations that we deem to be out of our control can trigger physiological, emotional, and cognitive processes that can lead to a heightened state of alert. And it's adaptive. For millions of years it has been potentially lifesaving to panic when a poisonous snake or other dangerous creature approaches us. Being able to flee (the "flight" in the panic-induced fight-or-flight response) can keep us alive. Most of us in the twenty-first century, however, don't encounter snakes every day; yet many of us feel fearful nonetheless.

In my case, my surroundings had become associated with potential threat; what was once just a neutral object, like a plastic container, had suddenly become inextricably linked with the trauma of my cancer diagnosis. Everything around me seemed ripe with possible harm—uncertain at best and treacherous at worst.

So what to do? How can we navigate stressful life events, rumination, and trauma triggers without additional suffering? So that futile worry thoughts do not derail our mental health?

Cue a look to ancient religions, particularly Buddhism. About thirty years ago, cognitive behavioral psychology researchers began to investigate the effects of centuries-old mindfulness-based practice on mental health. What they found is that becoming more present in the moment and nonjudgmental of our internal experiences—the basis of these ancient teachings—can lead to a reduction in distress.[4] It turns out that many of us can get stuck in a cycle of judging what may be normal human physical sensations (my heart is beating *too fast!*) or emotions (I *shouldn't* feel this way!) and then that judgment can result in panic or despair, above and beyond the original source of the anxiety.

Brains aren't computers. They are imperfect, spewing out assessments that are often nonsensical. And they can set off a chain reaction of conditioned responses to our current contexts, whether or not our responses are adaptive. Our thoughts can get in our way.

More than at any other time in my life, I needed to pull out my mindfulness-based tool kit to free myself from the "how did I get cancer?" rumination trap. I didn't know what caused my cancer. I didn't know if there was anything in my immediate environment that was maintaining its growth. I didn't know how much longer I had to live. I could choose to wrestle over these realities, or accept the inherent ambiguity, and sit still in the uncertainty.

12

FROM A TO C

How ironic to be diagnosed with breast cancer even though I have hardly any breasts to speak of.

As a preteen I watched as my friends went through puberty, sprouting hair beneath their arms, growing breasts, and getting their periods. Like them, I discovered fuzzy underarm hair and got my period, but I waited and waited for my breasts to more than bud. I bought a training bra—an aspirational purchase at best—and it made me feel a little less behind the crowd with my development, or lack thereof.

Some of the girls in my class had big breasts. The boys, all of a sudden, were transfixed by boobs. Their heads angled twenty-degrees downward as they walked through the halls, fascinated by mammary glands in all their nascent glory. I kept on waiting and hoping for something to happen. But my period was on a regular schedule, and there was still no sign of those things.

My mom, also not large breasted, shared with me that one day I'd be grateful for my chest. She explained that small breasts stay put, since gravity doesn't have as much to work with as we age. I was not reassured.

At some point in eighth grade I decided that the time had come, and I was going to have boobs. So I went to Bloomingdale's and bought a padded bra. Instantly my chest grew from an A cup to what I imagined must have been a large C. I don't recall if I made this purchase over a winter break, thinking that I could fool my classmates into believing that I'd had a hormonal surge, my breasts emerging over a few weeks' time. Or maybe I wore my training bra on a Thursday and then this padded bra on Friday—as if my boobs had grown miraculously overnight.

I do remember that I walked with confidence because of these new fabric breasts, my posture straight, head held high. I noticed boys noticing me, their heads tilted down at that twenty-degree angle, and I liked it.

Very soon after my new purchase, there was a weekend birthday party for a classmate. At the party, a girl from my class who had large breasts (real, I imagined) approached me and inquired with curiosity about my new body shape. She asked me, had I gotten any help from a push-up bra? No! I replied. I fervently denied any padding and insisted that my look was all-natural. I'm not sure how, but we ended up in the bathroom together, and she asked me to take off the bra so that she could inspect it herself. I had already committed to my story and was going to see it through. As I couldn't think of a way out of her challenge, soon enough, the bra came off.

I was caught. Between her thumbs and forefingers, the girl felt the impressive cone-shaped fabric mounds. My breasts, without assistance now, returned to their bud state beneath my shirt. I feigned confusion as the girl noted that I was, indeed, wearing a padded bra. Really? I replied. Humiliated, I played dumb and tried to convince her that I had no idea that this bra had added curves to my body.

I got rid of that bra, and over time, the fantasy of being big-bosomed faded away.

Many women diagnosed with breast cancer feel enormously protective of their breasts, which represent femininity, infant nourishment, and sex appeal. Though I mourned the loss of being able to breastfeed Siena, in all other respects, I was furious with my breasts and wished that I could rip them off my chest. They had mostly been a source of aggravation, first for their disappointing size, and then, as an omen of death.

Since I never ended up getting a lumpectomy or mastectomy, I do not know what it feels like to have my breasts taken away. Perhaps I would have wanted to safeguard them from surgical removal from my body, or grieved for my own flesh once they were gone. What I know for certain is this: I was wrong about my breasts playing a teeny tiny role in my life.

13

HELLO, MENOPAUSE

Prior to my diagnosis, my knowledge of cancer treatments and their effects was limited to depictions on TV shows and in movies—not the most reliable sources of data, especially when it comes to medicine. Before beginning treatment, I sought to educate myself about side effects in hopes that I could prevent or reduce the potential discomfort or, worse, a full-body breakdown. Since chemotherapy kills both healthy and unhealthy (cancerous) cells, all of me needed to be prepared for the attack. So I devised coping strategies with the guidance from the hospital staff, books (*Pretty Sick: The Beauty Guide for Women with Cancer*, by Caitlin Kiernan, was especially helpful), and a bit of trial and error on my end.

To protect my skin, I moisturized twice daily with cream specifically made for dryness related to medical treatment. I kept showers brief, lukewarm, and stopped using a loofa (too irritating). I initiated whole body oil applications at least twice per week, switched to sensitive skin deodorant and body wash, and applied super thick face and hand moisturizer. My skin remained crack-free and relatively hydrated during those months.

I applied nail cream at night, and though my nails didn't turn yellow or break off, my cuticles disappeared and created a gap between the nail bed and skin of my fingers. It was typically only uncomfortable while washing my hands or showering—a peculiar sensation to have water collect under a flap of skin that is meant to be sealed.

After every snack or meal I used a dry mouth oral rinse to help protect my teeth and gums. I carried a small bottle of it with me wherever I went so I could slip off to rinse in the restroom if, for instance, I was out at a restaurant. I used a gentle toothbrush with super soft bristles to avoid irritating my sensitive gums. I did not get any mouth sores.

Eating food became a strange experience often devoid of any pleasure. Sometimes, when I took my first bite of a meal—especially bread—I felt as if I were choking. I wasn't—it was the sensation of food getting stuck in my throat from dysphagia, or difficulty swallowing. After the first few times, I got used to this strange start to each meal.

I avoided eating my favorite foods on treatment days for fear that I would start to associate them with the chemotherapy, which could result in developing a food aversion. My fail-safe chemo meal was a muffin or turkey sandwich. Bland, simple. I sucked on all-natural candies during chemotherapy to help remove the metallic taste in my mouth. And I kept those lozenges with me at all times because the metallic taste would emerge even when I was not receiving treatment (water, especially, tasted like metal). I was lucky that I did not experience significant nausea and was generally able to eat most foods, even if they didn't taste like anything.

I was always fatigued, which is not the same as tired. After a full night's sleep, a tired body feels rested and restored. But no matter how many hours I slept, during the day and at night, sleep did not necessarily increase my energy. My bed beckoned me constantly, and I heeded her call to rest, rest, and rest some more. It felt as if the vitality had been sucked out of me, like when Ursula, the Disney sea witch, draws the voice out of the Little Mermaid. Simple conversations felt like marathons, depleting my body's energy stores. I read that exercise could help—but my being confined to a walker nixed that idea. Instead, I binged on TV shows I had not yet seen, like *Game of Thrones*.

My joints would feel as if they were locking up, particularly in the mornings when I started moving again after having been still overnight. I had to gently ease into my movements, which were stilted and lacked fluidity, especially when getting out of bed.

Constipation became a daily battle. I took an impressive array of medications to combat the opioids' stalling of my digestive functioning and the resultant stomach distention, but to no effect. In a state of severe discomfort and desperation, I donned plastic gloves and literally put my finger up my anus to manually remove the stalled shit from my bowels. One of my friends from high school, now a gastroenterologist, refers to this rectal clearing euphemistically as "pearl diving." I found no pearls, but I did find relief.

All this seemed necessary at the time, though, looking back, I can recognize the extremes to which I went trying to care for my body, which no longer knew how to care for itself.

What I was not prepared for was the abrupt cessation of my reproductive system. Chemo had effectively shut down my

ovarian functioning in one immediate assault, resulting in menopausal symptoms that are usually experienced gradually over
years. After having just given birth to a baby, my body must
have been mightily confused about what the hell was going on.

Every cancer patient has a different experience with chemotherapy. For me, the night sweats from the chemo-induced
menopause were the most challenging to contend with. My bed,
always a place of refuge and healing, became a space in which I
felt helpless and out of control. I started to dread the impending
arrival of nighttime because I knew that I was in for the inevitable doozy of a night's "sleep."

Within a couple of hours of shutting my eyes, I would wake
up, drenched in sweat, as if I had just dived, clothes and all,
into a bathtub full of water. The sheets, pillows, and quilt
were also soaked. Remaining in bed—freezing, shaking, teeth
chattering—was a terrible option. Though I knew that getting
out of bed would be, at least initially, even more uncomfortable.
As the cool air from our bedroom hit my skin it felt like a million little icicles were cutting into me, all the way down to the
inside of my bones.

I began to develop a nighttime routine: carefully creep out
of bed so as not to disturb Derek; move slowly with my aching joints and shaking body; breathe deeply through the sharp,
frigid sensations on my skin; grasp my walker to make my way
to the bathroom. Undress. Dry off with towel. Hang up soaked-
through clothes over shower curtain rod. Change into new pair
of clean pajamas. Make my way back to the bedroom, lay a dry
towel down on the bed so that I would not get soaked again
from the wet sheet below. Arrange myself back into bed, knowing full well that I would repeat this process at least another
three times before morning.

I discovered menopausal pajamas and sheets that reduced some of the wetness (so that I didn't need to wring out the liquid from my T-shirt anymore, for example), but the dark hours remained a conflicted time of rest and distress.

When my oncologist suggested that I start acupuncture to help with my side effects, I set up weekly appointments. I'm no expert on acupuncture, but I started with an open mind, hoping for some relief. After several weeks, my night sweats became less frequent (one to two incidents per night instead of four or five) and my achiness and pain started to decrease. I can't say with certainty that the acupuncture caused my symptom relief, but I can say that I have continued with acupuncture to this day.

The treatment side effects, though clearly unpleasant, were somehow bearable because they were evidence that the treatments were at work. My body was responding to the agents with unequivocal side effects—so maybe the chemo and immunotherapy were also invisibly decreasing the cancer cells, too?

14

'TIL DEATH DO US PART

Derek and I met at the beginning of my senior year in college. I had taken note of this handsome man around campus and at the local supermarket, but my friend Kat had sort-of-dated him, so I considered him off-limits. Since there were a lot of women and few straight men at my college, romantic relationships could get pretty incestuous, pretty fast.

On a Friday night, I was at the local bar called the Black Swan, for some reason by myself. I was friendly with the bartenders, so I imagine that I was probably hanging out with them. I noticed that Derek was playing darts with friends in the back of the pub. It wasn't long before he made his way to the bar to order another drink. He sat on the stool next to me and started talking about being from Brooklyn and studying literature. I told him that I was a painting major and a Manhattanite. He was a little eccentric and had me laughing. We ended up dancing to The Clash or some other alternative 1980s band, Derek swinging me around the dance floor. Then he kissed me. And it was a good kiss.

Early in the morning the next day (I swear all we did was kiss!) I walked back to my house, which was just a stone's throw down the road from the bar. I was guilt-stricken. I shouldn't have flirted with Derek. I certainly shouldn't have kissed him. What would Kat think? She is in a serious relationship with another guy, I thought, and is one of the most chill people I know. But who knows, maybe she'll be pissed anyway?

Upon waking on Saturday, I spoke with Kat on the phone (she was visiting her boyfriend for the weekend) and told her about the kiss. Her immediate response was "That's great! Derek's an awesome guy!" Oh, sweet relief—I had somehow gotten out of that one unscathed! Kat was genuinely supportive of our relationship from day one and has been to date—a full twenty years later.

Having been given permission to date Derek, I accepted his invitation to his house party the following weekend. Even though it was only our second quasi-date, Derek linked arms with me as he introduced me to his friends and older brother, clearly indicating that I was his romantic interest. I had butterflies. I knew that we were getting serious when he told me, about a month or so into our hanging out, that for his birthday present his mom had given him a gift certificate to take me out on a nice date in New York City. So he had told his mom about me!

I was falling in love with him.

Derek had a ruggedness about him. He grew up in Brooklyn and upstate New York—and had the perfect mixture of city boy/country boy in him. He was also super smart. I marveled at his brain as he described his college course on chaos theory, his passion for books and learning on full display most of his waking hours.

There was also an adventurous unpredictability to Derek that I found incredibly sexy. His behavior was in striking opposition to the cautious "always be careful!" messages I had received from my protective parents throughout my city-bound childhood. Soon after we started dating, he took me and his two guy friends Jared and Eamon to a ravine nearby in Hudson, New York, and both he and Eamon leaped off the edge of an impressively high cliff into the water hole at its base. Jared and I looked on in disbelief, our feet glued to the earth with no intention of moving, let alone jumping. After swimming around, his head just a tiny speck in the water far below, Derek climbed free-style up the rocky cliff as if it were no big deal.

Derek was tall, with defined, broad shoulders and toned arms that I imagined could easily swoop me up in the air like I was a lithe ballerina. He had large blue-gray eyes, a strong brow, and eyelashes, eyelashes, eyelashes. A chiseled jawline and full, kissable lips. His dark, messy hair conjured a 1970s-style shag.

There was also a kindness and sweetness to Derek. I could see that he was a loyal, dependable friend. He had good character— and even though he had his wild college antics, at the core he was steady and cared about doing right by people and the world at large.

A few months into dating we were at my house, lying on my bed together, when Derek started shaking slightly and lost all the color in his face. Was he OK? I wondered if he was going to be sick. After remaining silent for a few moments, he mustered up the ability to speak, and told me for the first time, "I love you, Sarah." I had never seen him nervous before. His vulnerability in the context of sharing his love for me enlarged my heart beyond measure.

We were the same age, but Derek was a year behind me at

college. He had deferred college for a year and spent half of that time painting houses, and the other half using the money he had saved up to travel to Spain, Thailand, and Ghana. After I graduated, we entered a long-distance-relationship phase as he finished up school and I bartended in New York City.

During his senior year, there had been one twenty-four-hour period in which we had broken up because of the physical distance between us. We were both in pieces: I sat in a chair and cried in that same spot the whole day; meanwhile, Derek was unable to move himself from his bed. We quickly decided to get back together and have been ever since.

We supported each other throughout it all: the partying; transitions; not knowing what to do with our lives professionally; trying to figure out how to be actual adults. Our relationship survived all of those bumps along the road, and now, after two decades of coupledom, we look back and feel as if we grew up together.

Once we started talking about marriage and the rest of our lives, we would smile as we imagined growing old together, toothlessly grinning, sitting side by side on our (fantasy) house's back porch, our grandchildren playing in the garden. Our skin wrinkly, bodies shrunken, our movements slow. Perhaps we would be physically unrecognizable versions of our earlier selves. But we would know, deeply, who we were, and how far we had come, still together, still side by side.

I had made a promise to Derek. I promised to love him forever. I promised to take care of him and grow old with him. Derek and I had made plans, and now I was fucking them up royally.

I was fixated on the thought that my being ill was such a raw deal for Derek, and that he had made a huge mistake in choosing me as his life partner. My guilt was so overwhelming that I implored him to leave me, to take the girls, in order for all of them to live their lives more fully. I wanted to protect them from what I knew would be the excruciating pain of watching me deteriorate and ultimately die an untimely death.

Derek, in his consistently calm demeanor, tried to assure me that I was crazy to think that he was going to go anywhere other than where I was. He told me that we were in this together, fighting the cancer together. That the cancer was the fuckup, not me.

I don't know how he was able to stay so steady with me. Derek's strength was staggering. He devoted his "paternity leave" to caring for me, and when he wasn't tending to me or our children, he was reading books about cancer or would be out running in Central Park. On his runs he allowed himself to completely break down in tears. Derek sobbed as he ran around the reservoir alongside strangers, surrounded by nature and fresh air instead of the stagnant air of a hospital room or cancer-patient bedroom. His eyes were bloodshot and puffy by the time he got home. But he always came home.

15

AN UNWANTED BODY

As a pregnant cancer patient, I had felt a fierce, instinctive protectiveness of my body; to keep my unborn baby safe, to let him or her continue to develop and grow. I held my belly tenderly and ran my fingers in circles around it, hoping my touch could somehow bring comfort to my little person, whom I feared would be taken from utero too soon. My pregnancy took center stage; its impressiveness was impossible to miss. The cancer, in its invisibility, was relegated to the background.

My relationship with my body changed dramatically after I gave birth to Siena and then discovered that the cancer had spread to my liver and bones. I felt disgusted. How could I be infested with this sickening, insatiable disease? It felt like there was no part of my body that belonged to me anymore. Instead, I was held captive by a terrifying, silent killer. I wanted to somehow trade myself in for a brand-new, healthy body.

Though many of us have complicated relationships with our bodies, we typically trust in their capacity to manage difficult situations. After a trauma, especially a disease like cancer, however, the body is no longer an ally; our brains, seeking to make sense of what has happened to us, cast it as the enemy. Such a traumatic event can activate the body's flight-or-fight reaction, and those physiological experiences may become *classically conditioned*, or unconsciously linked, to fear.

For example, after a traumatic event, an avid runner may regard exercise-induced increased breathing and heart rate as an indication of looming danger. These *interoceptive*, internal body sensations—your heartbeats, your breath—alert the now highly-sensitive-for-threat brain that you are not safe, and back into fight-or-flight you go. Your body was not in control during the traumatic event and continues to feel uncontrollable after the initial crisis has subsided.

Like a hammer to glass, trauma shatters our previously held assumptions that the "world is basically safe," that "extremely bad things won't happen to me," and "I'll be able to cope with any problems that come my way."[1] The formidable task of meaning-making in daily life requires that your basic, preexisting beliefs be grappled with and significantly altered, which is no easy task.[2] Although you are no longer in immediate danger, a new challenge takes its place post-trauma: incorporating the horrifying traumatic events into your understanding of yourself and of the world.

Not surprisingly, this period of traumatic response is often marked by intense emotions including shock, confusion, dread, horror, shame, numbness, guilt, and disgust. But perhaps most of all, you feel betrayed. The trauma violated your implicit understandings about yourself and the world: both, in utter defiance, have broken a tacit agreement of lifelong protection from harm by fundamentally failing to keep you safe.

When I entered this stage of trauma recovery, I thought of

myself as a lemon, no better than my parents' 1996 stick-shift Saab convertible that they continue to drive despite its being reliably unreliable. Even at a mere ten miles per hour, a blinking red light prompts the driver to shift up, the car demanding to be in fifth gear at all times. (I think it would combust if it ever made it into fifth.) The Saab routinely breaks down and leaves the driver stranded at the side of the road.

Quickly after starting treatment, I, too, was forced to slow down, with my damaged bones and walker, despite my yearning to run—to shift into fifth gear. Couldn't I ask for a body upgrade, trade in this lease for the newest model? I have so much left to give as a mom, a wife, a daughter, a professional, I told myself. But, in its betrayal, my body couldn't care less about my plans. The cancer had made its home in me; whether I approved of its residence there was entirely irrelevant.

It's not that I avoided mirrors, but what I saw in them was so unfamiliar that I was unable to fully integrate the notion that the person staring back was *me*. Fresh scars on my chest wall and neck from the central line port placement, the port itself protruding from my upper right breast area like a goiter. A little farther down my torso was the new C-section scar, red and bumpy. Baseball-size blue and purple bruises on my arms where I had initially received IV chemotherapy treatment followed by Heparin (the bruising culprit), an anticoagulant. My swollen uterus, my stomach distended from the near cessation of my GI tract, and more weight on my bones than I had ever had. My face, swollen from medications, pale-white and speckled with a pink rash, dark circles beneath my eyes. It was as if I were in a carnival house of mirrors—I did not recognize who that distorted person was.

In clinical psychology, we refer to traumatic stimuli (such as interpersonal abuse or natural disasters) as external triggers of internal distress.[3] Looking back, survivors can often recognize their primal drive to fight or escape their terrifying circumstances. But what happens when the source of trauma—that threatening stimuli—is your very own body?

The months of being poked, prodded, injected, cut open, and otherwise clinically examined by oncology professionals had resulted in my associating touch with cancer. That was until I had my first appointment with Liat, my medical massage therapist, who moved her hands gently and knowingly along my skin, relaxing my tense muscles and mind. Her touch carried with it compassion and care, and that felt to me both foreign, and at first, perplexing. I wasn't used to feeling anything other than pain or discomfort, but Liat challenged my view of my body as all-bad. It was through her hands that I started to rebuild a relationship with my flesh, my muscles, and my bones. I started to respect again, little by little, this home of mine.

With prescribed opioids to manage my pain, I also started to attend physical therapy appointments. The hope was to increase my balance and reengage the muscles around my pelvis and right hip through gradual movement. I was told that it was unclear whether I would be able to walk again without assistance from the walker; what was clear, though, was that my bones would remain too weak and susceptible to fracture for me to attempt twisting my spine or bending forward—movements that, precancer, were fundamental to my daily stretching ritual.

This wasn't the first time that I had felt confined by my body. As an eleven-year-old girl, I had been diagnosed with a curved spine and was relegated to wearing a brace around my torso for twenty-three hours per day. A year later, my back still not straight, I underwent spinal surgery to correct the scoliosis. Rods were inserted alongside my vertebrae to correct the S-shape. Due to my fused spine, flexibility was never my strong suit—and certain stretches were out of reach, including touching my own toes.

It wasn't until I was in my twenties that I found joy in movement. And at that time, for some strange reason, I decided that I *really* wanted to be able to touch my toes. So every day, for exactly sixty seconds, I would hang my torso as far over my straight standing legs as it could go. At first, my fingertips hovered just above my kneecaps. After at least a year into practicing, all that hanging got me to where I wanted to go. My fingertips grazed my toes. What a moment of celebration! Touching my toes had become one of my greatest personal accomplishments—I felt proud of my determination and the ability to train my body despite its anatomical anomalies.

Hearing from the cancer hospital's physical therapy department that I would not be able to touch my toes—that was a true blow. I had worked so hard to reach my toes and the ground beside my feet. I had become a gym rat, an aspiring runner, and a (somewhat inconsistent) yoga practitioner.

I could accept using the walker in the short term. Today, tomorrow. The day after, perhaps. But was there truly no hope of returning to my previous level of physical strength and abilities? Life could just be different, I thought. So I won't be the athletic sort I had been before. No more hikes in the woods or up mountains. No more jogs along the Hudson River, the breeze caressing my exposed skin.

Taking taxis to doctor appointments in New York City became my short-term replacement for that feeling of freedom and fresh air. I rolled down the windows so the crisp fall and then biting winter wind would make contact with my face. I was tricking my brain into thinking that I was the one moving through space quickly enough to feel that brisk sensation upon my flesh, hoping I would eventually adjust to this new reality.

I appreciate, as I write these words, the extent to which my denial was at work, almost like it was a friend of mine. But by worrying about whether I'd be touching my toes and twisting my spine again, I didn't have to face the harder question: whether I'd even be *alive* a few years from now.

On my walks around my neighborhood, I had made friends with the octogenarians who routinely stopped me to comment on my walker and give me unsolicited advice about how to make it move more effectively, like adding tennis balls to the front legs. And even though Sophie and my friends had decorated my walker with brightly striped, zigzag tape to jazz it up, I was eager to be rid of it and move again without feeling elderly and frail.

As was true in most subjects I studied, I was a motivated physical therapy student. I did my homework. I practiced the repetitive lifts of my legs, over and over again, while lying in bed, tolerating the discomfort but stopping before the point of pain. Gradually, I started to notice changes in my body.

A couple of months into physical therapy treatment, Derek and I were walking home from a date night in our neighborhood (all outings were contained within a five-block radius). Pushing my walker along, I found that I was leaning less on its handles and was moving my legs with greater ease. I said aloud, "Honey, I think I may not need this walker for much longer." We both started to cry. The thought of being free from the walker—to no longer encounter the puzzled gazes of people looking at me, trying to understand why this young woman was so infirm—would, perhaps, help me no longer view *myself* as infirm. This was serious progress, and we were elated.

After a few more sessions, my physical therapist agreed to let me walk my first loop around the hospital's gym sans walker. Then she added obstacles. Looking left, looking right. Slowing down, speeding up. I didn't lose my balance with any of these tricks. I passed the test! I was told to continue to use the walker while walking the streets of New York City for just a bit longer. The crowds, the variability of the sidewalk's terrain, would put me at too great a risk of losing my balance and possibly falling. But the end was in sight.

By late December 2017, I had been given the green light to walk the city streets independently, with just my body to propel me forward and hold me up straight. I stored the walker deep into one of our closets, hoping never to see it again.

The newfound confidence in my body, in its willingness to respond to my cues, challenged my previous designation of it as oppositional. Perhaps we could get along, me and this body of mine.

GANESHA AND OTHER
TRAUMA TRIGGERS

"How are you dealing with all of this?" my friend Danielle asked.

"I actually feel emotionally steady most of the time," I replied. This was not a state I could have imagined had someone posed the hypothetical to me before my diagnosis: How do you think you would feel if you were diagnosed with Stage IV cancer?

In the middle of the crisis, I had defaulted to the mode of rational, task-oriented, problem solver, my version of "fight" as my nervous system activated the fight-or-flight mode. There was always another doctor's appointment to attend, something to *do* to fight the disease. I heard the words of my oncologist, "*Keep going,*" in my mind on repeat. I intended to keep going, to keep living, but I also started to mentally prepare for the worst-case scenario, which in my case was actually very likely.

I started to concoct a plan to write an article about my husband—a CV-like description of his personality, ability to love, moral and ethical integrity, loyalty, how devoted and fun a father he is, his brilliant brain. In my bizarre notion, I would somehow publish the piece about Derek and predicted that women would line up to meet this incredible man. I would then help Derek interview the women, to help him find a warm, loving new wife and mother to our children. It was my way of ensuring that Derek and my girls would be cared for. Somehow this fantasy provided a feeling of (albeit delusional) control, as I imagined I could reduce the suffering of those I love most.

I now understand why my emotions were less accessible to me throughout the initial days of diagnosis, extreme pain, losing the ability to walk, and then undergoing treatment. It was adaptive for those feelings to remain suppressed—I needed to focus on the most important goal with absolute tunnel vision: to fight the cancer. At its extreme, this coping style can engender "emotional numbing," or the inability to experience and express feelings.

But there were moments when my emotions snuck to the surface and then took over; and unexpectedly, I entered a state of trauma-triggered panic. I felt as if I were in the middle of an emotional explosion. Out of control. Crazed.

After any horrifying event, the mundane facets of our lives can become instant triggers for fight-or-flight.[1] Day-to-day reality is teeming with sounds, tactile sensations, sights, and smells associated with the trauma. For a soldier who recently returned home from war, a previously celebratory Fourth of July fireworks display may now trigger the brain into alert of nearby gunfire. In the brain's *hypervigilant* attempt to prevent additional harm, neutral life experiences and body sensations are reinterpreted as a signal of clear peril.[2]

One evening, Derek and I had just gotten off our building's

elevator and were in the hallway upstairs, about to enter our apartment. My routine was to steel myself over before crossing the threshold in order to present myself as strong for our girls. But that night, my warrior persona simply wasn't accessible. I started crying hysterically outside our door, I couldn't find any air and kept repeating, over and over again, "I can't leave my girls! I can't leave my girls!" Derek tried to calm me down and held me up, but even in his solid arms I felt like I was drowning, sinking ever deeper into an abyss of despair. Ultimately, the overwhelming emotions abated and settled after reaching their peak. And we entered our home, greeting our children as if nothing was amiss.

Prior to beginning treatment, my friend had given me a brilliantly green, small statue of the elephant-headed Hindu god, Ganesha. In Hinduism, Ganesha is the "remover of obstacles," the god of success. Praying to Ganesha before any new endeavor is thought to bring good luck. I was so touched by the gift—I have always been interested in Hinduism, and elephants are by far my favorite animals. I placed the Ganesha on my bedside table, always nearby as I rested and slept.

One night while getting ready for bed I glanced over at my Ganesha statue. One of his hands had broken off. There was the textured, jagged, exposed inside of the statue, a lighter, less brilliant green, where his hand had once been. I don't know how the break happened, and it didn't matter. Like the flick of a switch, my calm and composed mood vanished and was replaced by what felt like an emotional tornado of anger, terror, and despair. Sobbing uncontrollably, I cried out to Derek that it was not okay that Ganesha was broken. Clearly, the Ganesha statue had come to represent more than just a thoughtful gift from a friend. It had become a symbol of hope, my metaphorical protector, and now he, too, was in pieces.

It was the first of January 2018. A new start. And hopefully a better year ahead. Derek, Sophie, and I were on our way to our local pizzeria for an early dinner. I had spent the previous week without my walker, roaming the streets, cautiously taking each step so as not to trip and risk falling. Derek and Sophie were a little ahead of me, and I picked up my pace to be beside them. And then, my shoe got caught on something—maybe a crack in the sidewalk—and I felt myself suspended in the air.

It was as if the fall was in slow motion. Though likely only a fraction of a second in duration, the moment seemed somehow elongated, like when you flip through the individual stills of a movie in book form.

There was nothing I could do to change the facts. I was falling. My fragile bones, which I had been told over and over again by medical professionals were ripe for breakage, were about to make impact with the pavement. I screamed because I knew—this fall could break my spine. My pelvis. Anything could shatter.

Derek turned around and yelled in horror, and then he and Sophie rushed to my side. I was still screaming.

Ordinarily, I carefully curate what Sophie sees and hears in my attempt to protect her from all things scary or disturbing. I am hyperaware of my own responses to challenging situations when my daughter is within earshot. Did I stub my toe? Don't make a big deal of it, Sarah, because you're modeling how to manage temporary discomfort with grace.

But on New Year's Day, Sophie saw and heard me wailing,

nonstop, for twenty minutes on that sidewalk. I had lost my ability to self-edit, to lower the volume, or to reassure Sophie that "Mama is OK." The fall and the pain were such intense trauma-triggers that my brain felt as if it had abruptly switched gears; in psychological terms, my prefrontal cortex (the center of rational thought) shut down and my limbic system (the emotional center of the brain) was firing with all its might. The sole thought, *my body is failing me, again!* was relentless as it repeated itself in my mind. I couldn't contain my reaction, not even for Sophie.

We New Yorkers are kinder than we get credit for. Several people on the street circled me immediately. One was a medical resident at Mount Sinai. Another a nurse. I stared up at them and said, "I have cancer," like that would somehow help them understand that this fall was serious. They stayed with me, there in the dark, on the pavement, until the ambulance arrived.

Once inside the ambulance, I kept howling, "I can't do this anymore!! What do you want from me?!? What do you want from me?!?" I didn't know whom I was speaking to. But I was looking upward, as if imploring the gods. I had reached my limit. Somewhere in the middle of my performance, I paused and apologized to the medic in the ambulance for my behavior. And then went right back to yelling my head off.

I was incredibly lucky. I had landed on my left hand, bracing the full weight of my body across my palm and four fingers. My hips were still solid. My spine, unscathed.

At the emergency room my ring finger started to swell. I managed to get my engagement ring off but the other wedding ring wouldn't budge. My finger turned reddish-purple from the pooling of trapped blood. Then began an assembly line of hospital workers, all with the goal of pulling this ring off my finger, over a knuckle that was clearly too large from injury to accommodate such a move. It seemed like a game for some of them. "Oh! I saw this once! We can tie string around the base of the ring and then pull it off!" And another, "Let's put petroleum jelly on the finger and then pull, that will work!" I screamed some more as they tried to wring the metal off me, and with each new "idea," more blood surfaced on my skin. Until finally, with resignation, they sawed off my wedding band.

I couldn't wear my wedding ring until the break had healed and swelling subsided. Given all that I had been through, that this was just a broken finger and a broken ring, it should have been the least of my worries. Yet every time I looked down and saw that brace, I was reminded of my fall. That ring finger had created a memory of the weight of the gold around its base, and now was naked without it. My wedding band, the representation of my relationship with Derek, was yet another integral part of me that had been stripped off and taken away.

So when the brace was finally removed, I decided to buy myself a ring. It was a skinny band with a single, tiny yellow gold circle. I donned my new ring and felt a little stronger.

Four months later, with the bone healed, rings repaired and sized up to accommodate my thicker, scar-tissued finger, my wedding band and engagement ring slid back into place. And upon their return, it felt like a fundamental part of myself had been restored. Though I continue to wear the tiny circle ring, but now on my right ring finger. It's a sweet, gentle reminder for me to take care of myself.

I still walk carefully, looking down for any uneven squares

of cement that aren't fully level with their neighbor. I do not look up at the towering buildings or treetops as I move through my city. I keep my eyes steady in a straight-ahead or slightly downward gaze. And give myself permission to stop walking to look at the sky.

SCANXIETY, ETCETERA

As a cancer patient (and a Stage IV one at that), I was slated to receive frequent PET/CT scans for the rest of my life. The results would indicate whether treatment was "working," which in the oncology world translates to no additional tumor growth. The goal was not necessarily to shrink the tumors but to put a halt to the rapidly dividing cancer cells. With each upcoming scan came the inevitable anticipatory anxiety: What will the results show? Is the cancer progressing? We in the cancer community refer to this phenomenon as "scanxiety."

But the fearfulness spread beyond the scans: to the blood draws that determined if my white blood cell count was high enough to receive another round of chemotherapy, or if treatment had to be postponed because my immune system was too weak to take on more of the toxic substance; to the weekly testing and then results of the cancer antigen levels in my blood; to hanging on to every word that my oncologist uttered, as if she were a god. What would she reveal today about my fate?

I became a helpless bystander as my body was evaluated.

At each weekly appointment with Dr. Dang, she examined my breasts and then the lymph nodes under my arms. She explained to me that if my breasts were a clock, my tumors were located at 11:00 and 1:00. By the time I started treatment, the 1:00 lump had grown to three centimeters with calcifications (dead, hardened cells that result from cancer growth) spanning at least five centimeters across my breast.

My initial biopsy examined my breast and lymph tissue for the presence and type of cancer cells, determining their Her2 positive status. But I was told that my liver cancer cells could differ in composition. It would be important to biopsy my liver to find out if additional treatments would be necessary to target the liver lesions.

During the "how to prepare for your liver biopsy" appointment at the hospital in early November 2017, I was asked about pain. When I denied any discomfort in my liver area, the hospital worker informed me, with no hint of empathy, that I would feel liver pain in due time. And that my stomach area would likely distend (beyond its already bulging state) from the cancer in my liver. Great, I thought. Thanks for the heads-up.

On biopsy day, I was relieved to have an emotionally attuned doctor who talked me, Derek, and my mom through the procedure. He pulled up the PET/CT image of my liver and noted where he would be collecting cells. My family was ushered out, and onto the procedure table I went. The doctor glided a sonogram-like wand over my stomach region. Minutes passed. No needles yet. Minutes more. Then the doctor said to me, "I can't find the cancer cells in your liver." He needed to speak with my oncologist.

Huh? Can't find the cancer cells in my liver? What the hell did that mean?

He returned from his call with Dr. Dang and said, "No liver biopsy today." Back in the waiting area, I told Derek and my mother the news. They were similarly mystified. We went home, baffled by the nonresult results.

My first posttreatment PET/CT scan was scheduled for the first week of January 2018, after completing the first half of chemotherapy and three months of immunotherapy. Until then, we would not know with any certainty how my body was responding to the therapies.

I was silently hopeful. The liver biopsy was confusing, yes— but it also awakened in me the notion that perhaps the cancer cells were being rightfully destroyed. Also, after only six weeks of treatment, I had been feeling for my breast tumor (as had become habit) and noticed that the 1:00 lump seemed significantly smaller—maybe even gone. Was that possible?

At my next appointment with Dr. Dang, she examined my breast. She no longer felt the lump there, either.

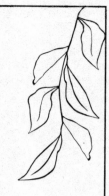

PART III

DISSOCIATION

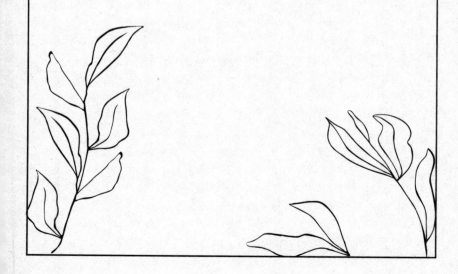

MY FAVORITE NAME IS NED

January 9, 2018. My parents, Derek, my brother (on speaker-phone from Idaho), and I awaited Dr. Dang, who had the results of my first PET/CT scan since receiving treatments.

Dr. Dang entered the now-familiar examination room holding sheets of paper. She brought them over and showed me the top page, which had a hand-drawn smiley face in the margin. With a wide smile of her own, she told me that I had achieved a "Complete Response" to treatment and that there was "No Evidence of Disease" (NED) in my body. That this was the best possible outcome we could hope for given my initial diagnosis. She described my "super-responder," NED status. Since my sensitivity to the treatment was so significant, we could decide whether to stop chemotherapy three months earlier than we had initially planned.

Derek immediately burst into tears. Before my cancer diagnosis, I could count on both hands the number of times I'd seen Derek cry. Since then, his eyes welled up frequently, not necessarily from sadness. Sometimes it was with gratitude for our support system; other times he seemed moved by his love for me and his girls. For that reason, I wasn't surprised to witness his unfiltered emotions pour out during the NED results, but I was surprised that I wasn't able to access those emotions myself.

I remember feeling confused and relieved, but mostly numb. I don't remember if I cried. I don't recall my other family members' reactions. Even though this was clearly outstanding news, I felt strangely detached, reminiscent of when I got the initial PET/CT scan results indicating aggressive, metastatic cancer. Nor did I comprehend what the results meant or this new vocabulary of NED and Complete Response. The cancer was gone? Or just that the PET/CT scan wasn't able to detect it in my body anymore? Had I in fact been cured? I no longer had cancer?

Dr. Dang explained that despite my NED status, there was still microscopic cancer "dust" in my body that a PET/CT scan cannot detect. I had not been cured; I would need to continue immunotherapy for the rest of my life in order to hopefully hold the cancer at those undetectable levels.

Though I couldn't identify it as such at the time, this emotionally frozen state was one of the many faces of my dissociation phase of recovery. Dissociation can be an adaptive response during a threatening situation, but if it persists long after the immediacy of the traumatic incident, it can lead to harm.[1] For those who continue to experience prolonged dissociation symptoms, the alteration in attention, memory, and awareness can interfere with what were once relatively straightforward activities such as reading or conversing with friends.[2] The fog of dissociation envelops the lived experience in which there is no past, present, or future and often results in a person appearing to be daydreaming.[3] In an inward collapse, there is the loss of psychological contact with people, the world, and the self. And at its most extreme, dissociation can dull the senses and interfere with detecting important safety cues in the environment, resulting in the potential for revictimization.[4, 5] This detachment from reality is a hallmark of posttraumatic stress disorder, with one study demonstrating that the vast majority (84 percent) of patients with PTSD struggled with dissociation.[6]

In my emotionally numb, intentionally ignorant-to-statistics state, I did not understand how atypical my results were. Later that week, my brother informed me that in the Cleopatra Trial, only 5.5 percent of the patients with my diagnosis and treatment plan achieved NED, and that was measured at six months' follow-up, not at my current three.[7] So the fact that my body had responded completely to treatment, and in this breakneck time frame, was nothing short of extraordinary. I had yet again become a statistical outlier—but this time, it was a statistic that I could celebrate.

Though I didn't feel celebratory. I remained mostly bewildered. In the days following my NED achievement, I felt like I had been thrust into a mysterious limbo between living and dying. At the time of my diagnosis, I was actively dying. No question there. Now, was my body closer to living, if there is a life-death continuum? On the one hand, my oncologist had told me that my body did not show any detectible cancer. On the other, I still in fact had cancer, and the treatments that I was receiving could stop working at any time. Apparently, cancer cells, like bacteria, are able to adapt. If my cancer cells figured out how to mutate and no longer remain sensitive to my immunotherapy agents, the cancer would invade my flesh and bones once again.

Entering into the coveted group of NED for metastatic breast cancer patients also came with downsides. Since we are a rare breed, there is scant research about our long-term prognosis. At the time of writing, I still have not been able to find statistics about survival rates among our group or an average time frame indicating when the microscopic cancer cells proliferate and, once again, spread throughout our bodies.

Dr. Dang said it was up to me whether to continue with chemotherapy or not. The concept of stopping—the chemo and side effects—was exhilarating. I had so wanted the medicine coursing through me when the tumors were its intended destination, but now I was loath to continue taking these toxic chemicals, which would also attack my remaining healthy cells. So my initial reaction was to proceed with chemotherapy that afternoon (as I had been slated to receive treatment after my appointment with Dr. Dang), but it would be my last dose. As we discussed the matter further, however, we decided that I would get chemo that day and then we would reconvene the following week to consider the next steps. My family and I needed more time to process the astonishing test results.

19

BUZZ OFF

As I grappled with whether to continue with chemotherapy, I found myself fixated on a particular side effect. Vinorelbine, the chemotherapy agent I ended up receiving after my allergic reaction to Taxol, typically does not cause baldness. But it can cause hair loss. It wasn't until two months of chemo that my hair started to fall out. I would wake up and see my pillowcase blanketed with my recently shorn, two-inch-long hair. And all of a sudden I started to lose it by the handful.

I was disturbed that I was thinking about my hair. When the assumption was that Taxol would be my chemo, I had made the firm decision to become bald. But when I learned that Vinorelbine would not cause baldness, I allowed myself to become protective of my hair and eyebrows. Vanity—of wanting to keep the hair that I had left—was an uncomfortable variable that I knew was impacting whether I wanted to continue with chemotherapy.

I planned to wait until my next appointment with Dr. Dang and make the chemotherapy decision with her guidance at that time. I tried to steady myself in a place of impartiality, weighing both the pros and cons equally, in the days leading up to the appointment with her.

In a rare break from the fatigue and the cognitive fogginess, I was able to get myself to the gym. I had recently started a physical therapy–approved exercise routine, including an upper-body ergometer and recumbent bike. I wore rubber gloves to avoid contracting illnesses, given that my immune system was compromised from chemotherapy.

In the aftermath of a trauma, a seesaw-like phenomenon, though not a playful one, may ensue in which there is an oscillation between the terror or fury of reliving the trauma on the one side, to avoidance or dissociation on the other.[1,2] That day, on the recumbent bike, my hair seemed to be falling out of my scalp every few moments, landing on my bare arm or inside the front of my T-shirt, producing an annoying, tickling sensation. I tried to retrieve each of the fallen hairs with my gloved fingers. After ten or so minutes of hair-removal-interrupted biking, I became enraged with trauma-fury—an emotion that felt foreign to me. My jaw jutted forward, my forehead furrowed. No more of this, I thought. And I abruptly dismounted the bike, made my way out of the gym, and found myself at a hair salon around the corner.

Buzz it off. Take it off, I said. I don't want to see it, to feel it, to think about it anymore. I sat in the black pleather chair as the stylist took the electric razor to my scalp. And I looked with disgust as the hair fell in clumps to the floor.

I had made a split-second decision to buzz off all of my hair so that I would no longer feel that nagging, unpredictable tickling, the repetitive reminder that I was not calling the shots. I also knew that by buzzing my hair, I could remove vanity from my chemotherapy "con" list and proceed with making a treatment decision based purely on medical considerations and not aesthetic ones.

But in doing so, I also lost my chance to prepare Sophie (and Derek). I got home, my black workout hoodie covering my head, and entered the kitchen where Sophie was hanging out with her babysitter. I told them, "I did something kind of crazy...," trying to make light of my rage-induced decision. I pulled my hoodie down and saw Sophie's look of shock and what resembled sadness. "I don't like it," she said.

I told her, I know it's a big change from what my hair looked like before. I asked her if she wanted to feel my new hairdo, but she refused. I asked her babysitter if she wanted to—and, recognizing that she was modeling for Sophie that it was okay to touch my head, she ran her hands through my buzzed hair. It felt good, she said. Thankfully, Sophie decided that she wanted to do the same. I bowed, and she stroked her little fingers along my scalp. I gave her a big hug.

That night, when I was putting Sophie down for sleep, she told me, "Mama, I want to get the same haircut you got." I told her we could talk about it in the morning, this being my favorite line to give myself time to think of an appropriate response to my daughter's more challenging queries. Come morning, she did not bring it up again. Whether she'd forgotten or changed her mind, I'll never know.

There had been times when Sophie, at age four to five, saw a man with long hair and asked me if he was actually a girl. I explained that hair length has nothing to do with whether someone is a boy or a girl. I reminded her that just because my hair is very short, I am still a girl. Yet she continued to come home from school with drawings of her and our family, Derek with his short hair, Sophie and her mama with long hair. It took over a year and a half after my buzz cut until she started to accurately represent my short do in her depictions of her family life. Though she continued to ask me when my hair would grow in again, because she said that it was "easier" for her to draw me with long hair.

Sophie was right on schedule developmentally. According to Kohlberg's theory of gender stability, five-year-olds often have not yet realized that cosmetic changes do not affect one's biological sex.[3] Although the specific gender norms of hair length may vary by cultural context, children can be especially rigid in their understanding of biological sex.[4] But now that Sophie is seven years old, she is able to identify a boy as still a boy even if he has a long ponytail and a girl as still a girl even if she has short hair. Since Kohlberg, the field of psychology has cultivated a more nuanced understanding of gender identity, too; recently, Derek and I more plainly explained the concept of gender to her—that our biological sex assigned to us at birth may not match that of our gender identity.[5]

But Sophie's questions, as childlike and innocent as they were, brought to the forefront my own desires to have long hair again. To pull it back from my face and twist it into a loose bun on top of my head. To have my husband run his fingers through the waves. I knew, rationally, it was just hair. And I knew, rationally, that long hair did not make me more of a woman. But I *felt* more womanly with long hair. And then the internal judgments popped up: Shouldn't I be confident enough with my female gender identity to not need an external representation of it upon my head? Why can't I break free of my yearnings to look more stereotypically feminine?

As parents, Derek and I have tried to shield Sophie from the bias toward all things pink and princess and the ever-present, nonsensical "girl aisle" in toy stores. We encourage her to play sports. We avoid commenting on her beauty and focus more on her inner qualities—her determination, focus, bravery, and kindness toward others. But starting in kindergarten, despite our best efforts, Sophie's favorite color shifted from orange to pink.

So Sophie loves pink, and I love long hair. Certainly, we've been socialized into these gender-normed preferences. Yet we still have the right to love pink and long hair.

I will grow my hair out long. And let Sophie choose which color shirt she wants to wear and which crayon to draw with. And I will continue to provide her with all of the colors in the crayon box to choose from.

20

IN THE HAZE

Now when I look back to when I learned about my NED, super-responder status, I can see clearly how unclear my reality was to me. By that January of 2018, the treatments and trauma dissociation symptoms had had their way with my cognitive functioning, and I was experiencing the mysterious "chemo brain," which so many of us cancer patients endure.

We don't know why these brain changes occur. Research has found that 45 percent of breast cancer patients experience "chemo brain" symptoms and that 36 percent continue to struggle with cognitive functioning six months after completing chemotherapy.[1] Cognitive impairment may intensify over the course of treatment as toxicity levels increase.[2] There is some thought that the cancer itself may play a role in cognitive symptoms, too. The short-term memory and executive function decline associated with chemo brain is enigmatic, and there are currently no evidence-based interventions to address the condition.[3]

For me, "chemo brain," likely in combination with trauma-induced dissociation, felt like viewing the world through a haze, as if there were a layer of gauzy fabric over my eyes. I constantly felt the urge to bring my hands in front of my face in order to part the fogginess, to draw away the curtains obscuring my view.

My short-term memory was seriously impaired—I could not remember conversations, names, and whether I had or had not completed a necessary task. In the words of U.S. poet laureate Billy Collins, it was "as if, one by one, the memories you used to harbor decided to retire to the southern hemisphere of the brain, to a little fishing village where there are no phones."[4] I frequently drew a blank when trying to express myself verbally (word retrieval issues) or would accidently use the wrong word entirely. For example, I would talk about buying groceries at the "shoe" instead of the "store." Interestingly, the wrong word typically shared the same first letter with the correct word.

Planning was especially challenging. Anything involving dates became an intricate puzzle. I squinted at my calendar, trying to focus as I arranged my schedule, rechecking my work. I routinely set up events for the wrong days. I would show up at an appointment that was supposed to take place the following week, or miss appointments entirely, even though I had "looked" at my calendar that morning. Despite my attempts to concentrate, it was as if my brain had significant blind spots and I would blank out information that was right before my eyes.

The day-to-day tasks that used to come relatively easily to me required a lot more effort. Previously enjoyable or simple tasks—like phone calls (even with dear friends), emails, and composing a shopping list—all seeped energy from my core. With my fleeting attention, I often found myself best equipped to stare silently at a blank wall. Minutes would turn into hours, and at some point I would snap out of the daze-like state. I would wonder how I could simply do nothing. Absolutely nothing. Without a trace of a thought. For hours on end.

All the while, my psychologist and I continued to meet weekly over teletherapy, saving me from having to travel to sessions. For the first time in my life, I had nothing to say in therapy. I couldn't muster the strength to speak. I just lay in bed, her gaze coming through the computer screen with empathy, concern, and what felt like love, for forty-five straight minutes. She stayed still and present with me in my silent fogginess. No matter how little of "me" would show up (cognitively or emotionally) from week to week, I could rely on my psychologist to therapeutically hold me in that haze.

Prior to my diagnosis, I was highly organized, efficient, and at times perfectionistic. I was a master at checking tasks off my to-do list with a laser-like focus. I got things done.

I don't know that person anymore. She is gone. It still gets in the way sometimes, my cognitive fogginess. I forget to do something, forget the request altogether, and let people down. But my new brain had also brought with it a gift. Completely unable to multitask, I now can only attend to a single activity at a time, which translates to being fully in the moment. I remember, precancer, the sense of needing to keep moving, to achieve, to catch up with that to-do list. Now, I am totally comfortable just sitting here.

Sometimes I wonder if my comfort in the present moment is an unexpected by-product of facing my impending, premature death. That my trauma has woken me up to a better way of living, of accessing gratitude in the everyday moments that create my life. Or maybe my presence isn't the result of some deep learning—perhaps I'm just too fatigued for my brain to worry as it once did. Worrying requires energy, and I no longer have the cognitive bandwidth to engage in a thought-juggling act.

At the next appointment with Dr. Dang, she and my family decided that I had had my last dose of Vinorelbine. The haze, fatigue, and myriad side effects had taken their toll. We would continue with the immunotherapy agents every three weeks to target the "microscopic cancer dust" that the PET/CT scan could not detect. But my body would now start its recovery from the toxic chemotherapy chemicals.

THE MIRROR

I am one of the few lucky ones. My body has thus far defied the odds of cancer progression, and worse, my death. Why I have been spared as opposed to the others who share my diagnosis is a mystery that at times haunts me.

Save for the few people whom we told over the phone, Derek and I revealed the news of my Complete Response over a mass email. The replies piled in, people writing about their relief and joy. I knew that I should have been floating in that sea of compassion and care, but all I could muster was the same detachment. During this dissociation stage of trauma recovery, it is common to experience a deadening of emotion or the feeling of dispassionate indifference. Individuals may also feel a surreal sense of being physically separated from their bodies, watching the trauma or its aftermath unfold from outside of themselves, often from a distance, perhaps from the ceiling or across the room.[1] For me, it was as if I were viewing the unfolding moments of my life from an airplane, taking in the aerial view from thousands of feet up in the sky; the reality below—

including my diagnosis and NED status—was a faraway blur, not totally real.

Perhaps surprisingly, dissociation can be adaptive during traumatic events.[2] When fighting or fleeing from a threat is impossible (being restrained by an assailant, for example), our nervous system initiates an emergency *freeze response*, in which the body collapses into a state of frozen paralysis.[3] Physical safety is unattainable, so the brain resorts to a psychological and physiological form of escape—an escape from conscious awareness. The incorporation of "freeze" in the "fight-flight" response ("fight-flight-freeze") more precisely describes our body's potential reactions in times of great peril. According to Judith Herman, the freeze response is one of "nature's small mercies, a protection against unbearable pain" in which "paradoxically, a state of detached calm" can dissolve "terror, rage and pain."[4] The surrendering response serves some mammals well, since predatory animals are less likely to detect immobile prey and, if detected, are less likely to attack animals that are perceived to be dead.[5] If an attack does ensue, the sensation of pain is diminished, and thus the targeted animal is spared from fully sensing their terrifying and painful demise.[6] We humans may misinterpret our passivity (during a physical assault, for example) as a sign of weakness, not understanding that, in fact, the freeze response is well outside of our conscious control.

Freezing is a form of dissociation marked by a numbed detachment from the present moment and a diminished awareness of your body and surroundings.[7] Our sense of time is distorted, often seemingly elongated or in slow motion.[8] Some of us experience a relatively harmless form of dissociation when driving and entering the dazed state of "highway hypnosis." You pull up to your garage and realize that you had "spaced out" while behind the wheel; you hadn't really thought about the turns, the stoplights, or much of anything at all, and have lost track of time.

If you don't recognize this in your own life, maybe you have observed this freezing response in animals—it's actually an involuntary and instinctual brain phenomenon in all mammals.[9] Perhaps you've happened upon a squirrel in the park and it abruptly halts its movement, transforming into a statue-like representation of itself. Or in the evening, you're driving along a country lane and spot an immobile doe at the side of the road. That cliché-but-real "deer in headlights" pose is her nervous system's activation of freezing in response to perceived danger.

When I told my medical massage therapist, Liat, that there was no longer evidence of cancer in my body, she was exuberant. Her emotions were an appropriate mix of surprise and elation. We had become so close over the two months we worked together; her hands had reconnected me with the good in my body and she had cared for me in a way that was immensely healing. Though despite our connection, I was disconcerted by her expressed emotions regarding my cancer status. In the days after our session, I realized that I had conveyed the remarkable news of my response to treatment in a very matter-of-fact, detached manner. Because I felt numb. The contrast between Liat's emotional reaction and my own was striking.

I encounter this phenomenon in my psychology practice. I am trusted with clients' painful stories and their emotions, which at times are almost imperceptible. As part of my therapeutic approach, I allow myself to express my own emotional responses to my clients' experiences, to model for them that feeling anger, fear, or sadness is not only OK, but is also often a normal response to a truly challenging situation.

Liat had become the sort of mirror I so needed—she shined a light on my emotional disengagement from my trauma experience.

But then came the guilt. The internal judgment of my detachedness. Why am I not jumping for joy? I *should* be exuberant, just like Liat, crying tears of delight at the news. After all, almost no one achieves NED status after being diagnosed with metastatic breast cancer. My lack of a strong emotional reaction felt like a betrayal to all of the women out there who die from their disease. Like so many others who struggle with dissociation, I found the experience highly unsettling and evidence of a personal failing.[10, 11]

I had every reason to be joyful, relieved, thrilled—*something*. But I couldn't locate my emotion states. They had been buried deep below, to a place where I could not find them.

22

THE GUILT OF SURVIVAL

Prior to one of my immunotherapy infusions, I sat in the hospital waiting area with my mom. The other patients around me are usually in their fifties or older, so I am typically the youngest one there. Sometimes people confuse my mother for the cancer patient simply based on her age. Because of this, I always notice when a younger-looking person is seated in the treatment waiting area, including the young woman who walked in that day, who looked about my age, with a man who looked like he might be her father, and sat across from me.

She looked pale and exhausted. I overheard her say to the man that she needed to put her feet up. I rose from my chair, found a small side table, and placed it in front of her, offering to help her to bring her feet up. She winced in pain as she thanked me.

I'm not sure how the conversation started, but she shared with me that she had been diagnosed with metastatic breast cancer a year and a half prior. She had tried multiple rounds of various chemotherapies, but none of them had worked for her.

The cancer had spread from her breast to her bones and liver. She moaned as she spoke about her liver pain, the aching in her abdomen. Sitting opposite each other, we were also at opposite ends of the spectrum of cancer treatment response. I was a super-responder, and she was dying.

Why? Why is she not responding to treatment? Why is this happening to her? And why on earth am I not experiencing the outcome that she is suffering? It's not fair. She deserves to live, just as I do. I could have just as easily been in her shoes, and seeing her across from me—the worst-case and most-common scenario for metastatic breast cancer—felt like a stab in the heart.

Typically, I enter the treatment infusion area with a smile on my face, greeting the nurses whom I now know by name. I have mostly positive associations with the treatment suite—it's where I was given a second chance to live. But that day, after I said goodbye to the young woman, I began to cry. A nurse, concerned, asked me what was going on. I told her about the sick young woman, and how unjust it is that she is unwell.

Like a roll of the dice, I was born into a family with means. I was raised in and then settled into a city that is known for having the finest doctors in the world. I have always had health insurance and access to excellent medical care. My parents are both alive, reside in my city, and are loving, devoted caretakers. My husband is my teammate—my true love. I have an incredible childcare provider, who adores my girls and keeps them happy and safe. My friends are kind, funny, and endlessly compassionate.

I know that these variables weren't causal factors in my reaching NED, but many people who get sick with cancer have nowhere near the resources that I have, which increases the burden of disease a thousandfold. They don't have health insurance or access to top-notch medical care or an attentive, empathic community. My cancer story is one of privilege, not just in my physical outcome to date—but in the many supports I have had in place from diagnosis to the present.

During the initial months of cancer, I was overwhelmed with gratitude for my life and the people in it. But my emotional repertoire vanished after chemo and the trauma-induced dissociation had its way with my brain. Guilt, always within reach, was the only emotion I could access. So, stricken with that unhelpful emotion, I judged myself for not being grateful *enough* about my NED status. Though the reality was that the cognitive fogginess and trauma-induced dissociation impeded my ability to feel much of anything. I was still in the haze, and didn't know if I would ever be able to get out of there.

23

PAST MEETS PRESENT

I was raised by a writer. My mother's golden Emmy Award shone proudly on our black piano; her novels, translated from their original language to be read around the world, filled our bookcases. Back when I was in high school, my mom and I sat in the windowed kitchen nook together as she marked up my essays, adding brackets around sentences that she notated as "awk" in the margin. She never expanded upon this declaration—what made my writing awkward, or how to fix it. Instead, she sat with me, ever-so-patiently, as I tried to figure it out. We spent hours upon hours poring over my writing. She instilled in me an appreciation of language, so much so that at times I have been compelled to stop and marvel.

Like the time when my mother taught me the meaning of a widow sentence.

As a narrative therapy psychologist, in a way I have adopted my mother's role as writing teacher, supporting my patients as they find the language to clearly tell their stories. And I have witnessed the benefits of narrative storytelling; by bringing language to our traumas, disjointed memories can find their place in our living memoirs. I've worked with many patients who start off treatment saying that they "can't remember" much of their trauma. And for good reason. Our minds try their best to avoid that which causes distress—the memories of pain, terror, or betrayal. Additionally, normal memories are thought to be stored differently from traumatic memories, which become "sensory fragments" with minimal verbal components, often experienced as perceptions, behavioral reenactments, or ruminations.[1]

When I decided to experiment with writing my own trauma narrative, I made a rough outline of the significant events associated with my cancer in chronological order: initial diagnosis, when and how to give birth to Siena, NED results, etc. Taking on the role of patient, I followed the same treatment plan as the narrative therapy approach I provided my clients, writing down a brief description of what would later be expanded upon in written or oral form.

Once I started writing, I was surprised at how quickly the early crisis days of my diagnosis and early treatments seemed to tumble out in a deluge upon the page. But when I tried to start writing about those days of staring at the ceiling, I felt stuck. I was puzzled because it was the dissociation symptoms that had propelled me to write in the first place. Though when it came time to write about this stage in my trauma recovery, it was as if the psychological haze of my past was clouding my ability to describe the experience.

I was back to that familiar staring scenario, though this time it was at my blank computer screen as opposed to the ceiling. But I remembered the writing lessons my mother had taught me—

the ubiquity of writer's block and its antidote of perseverance—
and I trudged on and kept writing.

Now, as I look back, I understand that part of my confusion
was related to the fact that I was almost finished writing the
story of my traumatic past. I had gathered the memories and
brought language to the initial diagnosis, when and how to give
birth to Siena, and the NED results, all clearly recorded in black
and white. My unsettled feeling was a knowing that, despite the
near completion of my trauma narrative, my trauma recovery
was not yet complete.

So I decided that I had more to write. My traumatic history
was now ready to meet the realities of my trauma recovery as it
unfolded in the present.

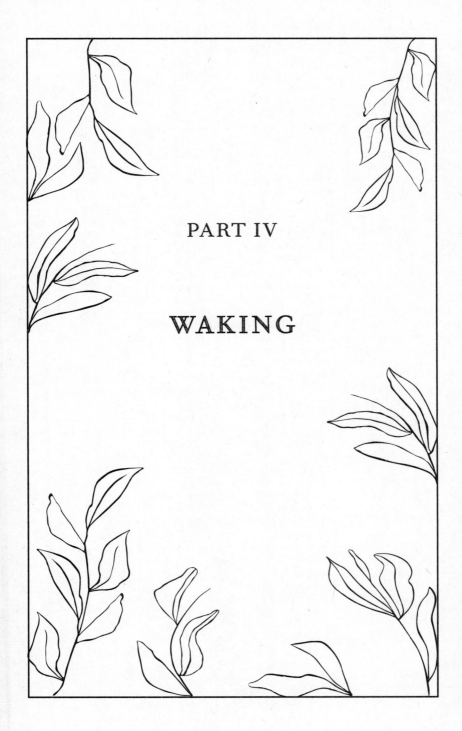

PART IV

WAKING

24

MOVING TOWARD RECOVERY

OK. I just fought for my life, and against the odds, I'm here. Now what?

I was told that I would be in recovery from chemotherapy for a year or two. My bones still needed to heal over from where the lesions had eaten them away. Hopefully, with physical therapy, I would be able to move again with relative ease, though the radiation site in my pelvis would likely be a chronic source of tightness and pain, reducing mobility. I would continue immunotherapy treatments (Perjeta and Herceptin) every three weeks. Frequent PET/CT scans and blood draws would keep an eye on the potential for cancer regrowth. Even though I was NED, I was clearly still a cancer patient, visiting the hospital multiple times per week to receive oncology-related services.

My postchemotherapy, emotionally traumatized brain was starting to wake up. The content of these new thoughts, namely, *What the fuck just happened?* played on loop as I attempted to start to make sense of the significant, terrifying events of the previous five months. I was in a state of bafflement, questions populating my mind, all with no clear answers. Do I embark upon living again? Assume that the cancer will not proliferate, and try to build myself back up to my previous, precancer self?

In the throes of dissociation, thinking, feeling, and sensory awareness are fragmented or nonexistent; the sense of self is lost, personalities erased.[1, 2, 3] But in this new stage of trauma recovery, the fog starts to part, time is set in motion again, and the shuttered mind and body start to let in the light of day, hesitantly. Emotions, body sensations, and thoughts—previously either entirely overwhelming or in absentia—are noticed again. Memories are no longer shrouded in a haze, and the traumatic event is at the very beginning stages of being incorporated into an understanding of the self, the body, and relationships. Though grappling with such horrifying facts requires a sort of wiping out of your history of beliefs. But like a writer staring at a blank page at the beginning of a new story, there is a budding sense of possibility.

For me, I poured this novel awareness and burgeoning potential into movement. Freed of my walker and full of newfound, albeit inconsistent, energy, I started to widen my radius of exploration beyond my bed. Physical activity had the added benefit of helping me direct my attention away from those ruminative, cancer-obsessive thoughts.

I also had a specific, incredibly meaningful goal. I was able to hold and snuggle little Siena and respond to her coos and facial expressions (almost always it was a smile) with ease. That was all Siena really wanted and needed from me in her early days. But Sophie, four years older than her little sister, was constantly on the go. I felt an urgency to regain my physical capacity, to return to the mom-daughter play that had been off-limits for so many months.

After I started walking again, I became determined to learn how to kneel down to the floor and stand back up so that I could engage with Sophie on her level. During those physical therapy sessions I felt baby-like, relearning the essentials of movement that I had mastered in infancy. I diligently practiced the lunge moves, repeating them slowly, until I was able to get back to where I had been so longing to be—on the ground beside my older daughter, in her world of imagination and creativity.

In February, after months of hard work, I was finally able to pick up Sophie again. We were both beaming with joy. Those parts of my body, around the waist and neck, had felt an emptiness without the weight of my first child resting her dangling limbs against me. But I got her back into my mommy nook and was overcome with gratitude that I could embrace my big girl again.

In the late spring of 2018, I continued to work on building strength and stamina, spending time at the gym or at home practicing exercises daily. Music had always been an essential part of my workout routines, and Derek had made me the best playlists, which invigorated me as I went on precancer runs throughout New York City. But it didn't occur to me to listen to his compilations postdiagnosis—I was still at the rudimentary stages of becoming physically active, and silence was my soundtrack of choice.

One day at the gym while I was on my way to grab the five-pound free weights, a song from one of Derek's old mixes came on over the speaker system, "O.N.E.," by Yeasayer. I stopped dead in my tracks. I remembered running along the Hudson River, back when we lived in Chelsea during our graduate school years, my feet hitting the pavement along with the song's beat. It was the second or third track on Derek's playlist, perfectly timed for when I had just found my stride after the initial jog warm-up. I remembered the feeling of the sun on my skin, the ease with which my body propelled itself through space. And I realized, as I broke down into tears, that song (and all the mixes Derek had curated for me) had become a soundtrack representing tenacity and freedom.

I had made enormous progress in terms of my movement, but I wasn't back there yet, able to run or feel a sense of empowerment in my body. And though I wasn't angry or necessarily sad, I continued to cry, standing there in front of the weight racks and bodybuilders. I didn't care who saw me—other people were the furthest thing from my mind. I gave myself permission to honor the meaning of the memories and emotions pouring out of me. I was starting to feel again.

25

CANCER-INDUCED ADOLESCENCE

Each time I passed storefront windows in NYC, I caught the reflection of a person with soldier-short hair, an oval body shape from having baby number two, and bloated from cancer treatment. It took me a moment to realize that this person was not a boy but a girl—no, a woman—and that woman was *me*. I continued to be amazed by my shock each time I met my reflection. Who is that? I don't recognize her. I don't know her. She is a strange stranger.

At the gym, my place of hope and healing, I found myself returning to the music I had listened to as a teenager. I was especially drawn to Liz Phair, who was a favorite during my adolescent period of angsty self-discovery. Why was I responding so deeply to Liz Phair? Earbuds in, I immersed myself in her voice, defiant and strong.

Out living my life again, I started to meet people who didn't know my story. They would ask my name, and I would swallow the response that wanted to tumble out of my mouth: "Hi, I'm cancer." But cancer was not my name. I was still Sarah. And

Sarah has cancer (or at least the NED varietal). I am Sarah, and I have cancer. I wondered if there would ever be a point in time when the word CANCER wouldn't be the only word on repeat, popping up in my brain like a broken record.

I am not alone in being distracted by thoughts that have nothing to do with the present moment. A study out of Harvard University found that we humans spend almost half of our waking hours with a "wandering mind"—thinking about the past, the future, or something that might never even occur—and unfortunately for us, this wandering often leads to unhappiness.[1] Having had a mindfulness practice precancer, I had tools to focus my thoughts on my current, in-the-now moments. But despite my best efforts to change the script in my brain, my inner monologue was mind-numbingly redundant. Indeed, at this stage of trauma recovery, thoughts related to the traumatic event are still at the forefront of the mind and predominate cognitions. No matter where I was or what I was doing it was more of the same: CANCER, CANCER, CANCER.

Cancer had eaten up my bones, and now it was devouring all of the space in my mind. It had become my primary, defining identity. I didn't know if or when I would be able to find the other parts of myself, or if they even still existed.

A trademark of being a psychologist is having endless curiosity about people. Living in a New York City high-rise provides me with momentary glimpses into the worlds of others. Riding up in the elevator with my neighbors, I start to wonder. Parts of their lives are hinted at during that thirty-second snippet of conversation with their friend, family member, or lover. The choice of attire, an expression on the person's unfamiliar face. He has a shopping bag in hand—what did he just purchase at the store? Favorite foods, a houseplant, or diapers? Each detail tells a story; I feel surrounded by living novels, rich and complicated and beautiful.

It was after 5:00 P.M., and the elevator was crowded with workers and kids returning home after a full day. An adolescent male towered above me; he must have been at least six foot four, lanky, perfect for basketball. Despite his impressive size, his face gave away an unmistakable boyishness. The mismatch brought on a surge of memories from my own teen years, of trying to find my own place in my body as it lengthened and grew, and attempting to keep up with its pace of maturity.

The boy was frustrated. His puppy brown eyes were wide open despite his weighty, dark, long eyelashes. He groaned in dismay as he saw the numbered buttons illuminated, indicating the stops en route to his higher floor.

"Ughhhhhh, I'm too *tired* to wait for all of these!" the boy moaned to his father.

A woman next to them (his mother?) said, "OK, OK," as if trying to calm the boy down.

"I'm getting out. I'm walking!" the boy announced.

The father looked at his son in disbelief, saying, "That makes *no* sense. If you're tired, why would you walk up ten flights of stairs?!?"

The woman intensified her OKs and then got off the elevator at the next stop (clearly she was not with these two—interesting that she tried to intervene). The boy looked again at the yellow-glowing numbers, and at the next stop, he grunted with indignation and stomped out of the elevator, hunched slightly by the weight of his backpack, his father left standing in the car, flabbergasted.

"I don't get him," he said as the elevator doors closed shut.

I laughed (a little too unrestrained, I fear) and shared, unsolicited, that his son was right on track.

I know the frustration the boy felt so intensely in that elevator. Of feeling trapped in his circumstance. The "get me out
of here" and "make this feeling go away" mentality. Adolescence can often feel like a never-ending ride in a cramped elevator to independence, adulthood, and emotional stability.
We're convinced that we're ready for the final destination, but
in reality, our emotions are too hot, our prefrontal cortexes still
underdeveloped. But we don't understand that yet. So we end
up being highly reactive, not-so-rational beings just trying to
negotiate our way through this period between child- and adulthood.

After my NED-designation, I felt thrust into a kind of second adolescence, which brought on that familiar feeling of
impatience. Although instead of existing in a suspended state
between dependence and independence, I was navigating the
precarious spectrum of sickness and wellness. I wanted to get
to the next stage in my recovery, but as in adolescence and its
corresponding biological, hormonal, and brain changes, I was
also at the mercy of my body.

Back as a teenager, I remember the volatility of emotions
and thoughts as I tried to figure out who I was. The normal
biological changes of adolescence resulted in my body feeling
unruly. So I seized upon ways to somehow take back the helm.
I experimented with clothing (punk, hippie, even a brief goth
phase), piercings, and dyeing my hair. I was, like so many other
adolescents, trying to build up my sense of self during what
felt like an internal tornado of instability.

Here I was again, so many years later, enduring those same

out-of-control feelings. My hormones were going berserk between giving birth and then being thrust into chemo-menopause all within the span of a single month. My body rapidly shifted from cancer proliferation to treatment-induced cancer obliteration. The disease's ramifications and treatment side effects yielded extreme unpredictability from one moment to the next.

I had a choice. I could continue to assume that the cancer would grow back at any time (as the odds favor that assumption) and hold on to the fear, vulnerability, and despair. Or I could pursue the more optimistic (though unrealistic?) line of thinking: NED was my new, and hopefully permanent, reality.

In a sudden rebellion—my version of walking up ten flights of stairs—I purged my apartment of all its cancer-related gear. Out went the menopause bedsheets, the dry mouth oral rinse, the sensitive skin electric razor, the children's books about mom with cancer—into a large plastic bag, and then down the garbage chute. The sound of the bag falling, tumbling down that black abyss, quieting with its rapid descent and landing with a thump atop the other discarded parts of people's lives, roused a satisfaction that I hadn't expected. My home was going to be a place to celebrate life. I would no longer assign valuable New York City closet space for Stage IV cancer stuff.

During this phase in my cancer recovery, my hair started to grow back, but this was not hair that I could recognize. There were oval-shaped patches of black, wiry hairs growing out of my head. A hairdresser told me that this was "chemo hair," and that I should continue to buzz it until the "nontraumatized" hair grew back in. So I buzzed and buzzed, waiting for the black patches to give way to the blond, soft textured hair that I'd had before. Instead, a reddish-iridescent hair came in next, the color of a bad dye job. I kept buzzing, waiting for myself to grow back.

After four months, a normal (for another woman), chestnut-colored hair grew in, uniform in color across my head, and smoother to the touch. My once blond wavy hair was replaced by brown curls, a new look for the new sort-of-postcancer me.

Amid all of this change I felt an unexpected impulse to tattoo my body and add piercings to it again. If I reflect upon that desire now, it seems to me that I was searching for a way to exert authority. I longed to do something that was intentional, and remind myself that I had some say over my body and how I presented it to the world. The fact that I could choose to change my appearance felt like a form of power. I'm the boss of you, body. You do what I say!

I didn't end up getting a tattoo or another piercing. But I started the task of rebuilding myself physically, mentally, and emotionally. Sometimes that entailed stomping around New York City, headphone volume blasting, as I listened to an angst-ridden, 1990s-era punk rock star.

26

RETURN FROM
MATERNITY LEAVE

In the second trimester of my pregnancy, I informed all of my patients that I would be taking three to four months off for maternity leave and return in the New Year. As it turned out, my leave started earlier than I had anticipated, as the cancer diagnosis preceded my due date by about seven weeks. Luckily, I had already discussed with my clients whether they wanted to continue with therapy (and if so, I had provided them with the transfer psychologist's information).

I had spoken with my bosses once I received the initial diagnosis in September 2017. Despite my attempt to present the cancer news in a composed and professional manner, tears streamed down my face and my voice broke as I relayed the facts. They were compassionate, kind, and assured me that my patients would be well cared for during my absence. I told them that I hoped that I would get back to work in January, as I had originally intended. My oncologist had told me that some women are able to continue to work while receiving chemotherapy—and I decided that I would aim to be one of them.

Once I learned that the cancer was metastatic, the original return-to-work time frame became glaringly unrealistic. I contacted my bosses to update them and revised my start date to March.

My level of denial—thinking that I would likely be well enough to return to work in March—was profound. But I held on to the idea of March with a tight grip. I love my job. It is a part of who I am. My clients and I had more work to do together.

When I learned of my NED status, March became a target that I could conceivably reach. But cognitively, I was nowhere near as sharp as I had been prior to treatment. Would it be ethical for me to return to work if my cognitive functioning was not at its previous level? Would I be able to provide effective psychotherapy now? Ever?

But I remembered that like a muscle, the brain can be strengthened through exercise. Years ago, neurologists believed that over time we lose neurons (brain cells) as we age, resulting in an irreversible decline in brain function. But now we know that this original theory is misleading. Neurons actually continue to generate well past their initial proliferation in infancy, childhood, and adolescence. This process is called *neurogenesis*, and it enables us to stretch and enhance our brain's faculties the more we keep it active.[1] Hence the recommendation for older people to engage in challenging mind games, like crossword puzzles, to help delay the onset of dementia and other age-related cognitive decline.[2] So perhaps my brain would be able to adapt to the challenges of clinical work after all.

In talks with my oncologist post NED, she assured me that I

was physically and cognitively able to return to work, but advised me to pace myself. I also had my two young girls at home and wanted to find a balance between work, spending quality time with Sophie and Siena, and tending to my ongoing medical care and self-care. I decided to start back at work two days per week, and resume psychotherapy with my previous patients only.

March arrived—and like some miracle, back to work I went. My hair was now buzzed short, I had dark circles under my eyes, and my face was pale. But with my white blouse and black pants work uniform on, I felt almost ready to be a psychologist again. None of my clients knew about my health crisis, that my extended "maternity leave" was actually a fight for my life. My patients understandably assumed that I had simply chosen to stay at home for the additional three months to care for my infant.

In the world of psychology we often reflect upon the notion of "disclosure." How much do we share about our own lives with our patients? In the more-Freudian style of psychotherapy, the goal is to remain a *blank screen*—that way, any feelings that emerge within the patient about the therapist are thought to be projections based upon the client's previous relationship patterns.[3] In order to facilitate this blank screen, some therapists ask their patients to recline on a couch, close their eyes, and free-associate, removing the therapist as a potential distraction or influencer as clients gain access to their unconscious realities.

I work differently in my practice. I face my patients, who sit upright (albeit in a very comfortable chair). I make eye contact with my clients. One of my treatment goals is for my patients to feel safe to lay bare all of their difficult thoughts and feelings, and to allow themselves to be seen and accepted by me, in all of their beautiful, human messiness. I am actively engaged during sessions, communicating through the power of language, non-verbal behavior, and empathic attunement. I am very much a human being sharing the therapeutic space with another human being.

There are inevitable hints about my personal life present in the sessions. For example, I wear a wedding ring. It's interesting when some people comment on it. One day a patient of mine announced "You got engaged!" even though my wedding ring had been on my finger for far longer than I'd been this person's therapist. Others scan me when they first meet me, trying to get a sense of my story. Some of my clients are surprised to learn that I have children. Another surmised that I had "about a dozen" kids. The meaning behind each patient's idiosyncratic viewing of me can lead to the exploration of deep interpersonal dynamics.

Not surprisingly, a major disclosure that is difficult to conceal is a rapidly growing belly. All of my patients knew that I was pregnant (with the implicit understanding that their therapist, in all likelihood, had sex!). Some incorrectly assumed that I was pregnant with my first child. The pregnancy itself was triggering for those who had experienced a traumatic pregnancy or delivery, and others were concerned I would soon be taking time away from caring for them to care for someone else—my baby. A mix of excitement and anxiety was a frequent, and normal, response to my pregnancy.

In anticipation of my return to work after giving birth to Siena and fighting cancer, I prepared for my patients' querying about what I perceived to be my dramatically different physical appearance: namely, the transformation of my hairstyle from long-blond to buzzed-brown. I sought out clinical supervision, meeting with expert psychologists to ask about how to manage my own anxiety about the possibility of my medical status taking over the therapy space, and made a plan of action. As is my usual approach, I would not bring up my hair or anything related to myself unless asked by the patient. Depending on the client, I would choose how much to disclose about why my look was so different.

In the past, there were never blatant indications that something challenging, let alone traumatic, was actively going on in my life. Now, it felt to me as if my trauma traveled with me wherever I went. I not only looked different, but I also looked ill, like a cancer patient. Was I far enough out from my trauma to appropriately respond to my patients' possible remarks about my appearance? Would I be able to remain calm and focused on the client's needs, and not get lost in my own emotional response? I worked hard in my own therapy to make sure that I was as ready as I could be to be present for my patients.

As I greeted them, each one inevitably commented on my new hairdo. I got a lot of "wow"s. One said that I looked "bad-ass." Another, while on our way to the session room together, said the following contemplatively: "I always think that when someone makes a big change to their appearance that something major is going on for them." His statement remained a statement as opposed to a question, so I indicated with a silent head nod and curious eyes that I had heard him. Once we were settled in the therapy room, the focus naturally shifted to him. But when I greeted another one of my clients in the waiting area, she looked shocked. Once in my office, she sat down, leaned forward in her chair, and said, "You had chemotherapy." She knew.

This was a patient with whom I had worked for years, who showed up early every week like clockwork. A writer, she is gifted with words, and we immediately found ourselves in a therapeutically rich relationship full of mutual respect, a love of language, and a dedication to psychological growth and learning. She was the first patient to notice that I was pregnant, before I had planned to bring it up with my clients. (I didn't think I was showing at that point—she knew better.)

There was another tip-off that something was amiss. Before I took maternity leave, this same patient asked me, earnestly, if there was a chance that I wouldn't come back to my practice after I had my baby. A fair question. I told her that barring anything unexpected, I would be back in January. That in addition to having a growing baby in my body, I also have a fire in my belly that propels me to do the work that I find both challenging and enormously gratifying.

Come January, ready to resume the work of therapy, she emailed me, asking about my return. I responded that I was extending my leave and would be returning to the office in March. She emailed me back that she hoped I was enjoying the extra time to bond with my baby.

Back in the office space together, I returned my patient's gaze and told her, calmly, that yes, I had undergone chemotherapy. She asked a few more questions, like the type of cancer (I said breast but didn't specify my stage). She asked me if my baby and I were OK now, and I told her, yes. As breast cancer is so common (one in eight women will be diagnosed with breast cancer over their lifetimes), and this patient is one of my older clients, perhaps it was easier for her to integrate this information without it derailing our treatment.[4] Once I assured her of my ability to care for her, we dove right back into our work together.

It felt like coming home.

27

FUNERAL MUSINGS

As a young child, I had a flair for drama, strong opinions, and unwavering (some may say rigid) notions about what I judged to be right or wrong. When my internal moral compass was challenged, I would not take it in stride. The phrase "You'll see! When I run away! Or I *DIE*!" rings a bell. My poor parents were the recipients of my irrational fantasies that in my absence, they would see the light.

On one occasion after being *blatantly* wronged and *completely* misunderstood (the majority of my childhood and adolescent thoughts belong in italics), I found refuge under my bed. I told my parents that I would be staying there until their minds had changed. What the slight was, I cannot remember. It may have been the time that I was no longer allowed to watch *The Simpsons* after my mom caught a glimpse of Homer drunkenly stealing money from one of his cartoon children's piggy banks to buy more beer. But Mom, what was Sunday night at 8:00 P.M. without *The Simpsons*?

I do remember the slightly cold black-and-white-tiled floor—
like a chessboard—and my little six-year-old body enclosed in
my not-so-secret hiding space. I stared out through the holes of
the white, intricate lace bed skirt, which landed an inch above the
ground. I could see the outside world, and its potential, through
that inch of unobstructed space. But I stayed put.

My father appeared, and leaning against my bedroom's
doorframe, he calmly attempted to reason with me. "Sar, you're
painting yourself into a corner . . . " while I covered my ears
with my hands and silently intoned *La la la* to block out his
patient and loving words. He'll see! I thought. At my funeral,
they'll know that they made the biggest mistake. They'll all be
crying and feel so bad for what they've done!

That funeral fantasy felt like the ultimate revenge. And then
I would tilt my small head and squint my little eyes and wonder
. . . who would be there? What would be said? I imagined a sea
of people all in black, mourners huddled together, broken to
pieces without the all-important *me*.

In a dark, twisted reality, my cancer diagnosis gave me a preview
of what my funeral might actually look like. I was surprised to
see the turnout. The notes poured in with mini eulogies, full of
warmth and kindness, my under-the-bed, childhood yearnings
met. Wanting to do something tangible for me and my family,
my whole network, which felt like it was growing daily, rallied
to take care of us.

My friend Lauren suggested that she set up an online "meal
train" so that weeknight dinners would be dropped off at our
apartment. I remembered trying to eat when Sophie was a
newborn—grabbing a slice of bread or tearing off a piece of ro-

tisserie chicken, quickly stuffing it in my mouth for some fuel. It had to be fast and efficient. Absolutely no home cooking took place those first few weeks of motherhood.

Derek and I initially resisted the idea of the meal train. We didn't want to inconvenience people or make them feel obligated to spend time and money on our family. But we ultimately decided to give it a try. And it was, without a doubt, one of the best decisions that we made during my illness.

Lauren set up the website and sent out an email asking people to sign up for a time on the train schedule. Within forty-eight hours, all slots had been filled with names of people whom I knew and loved. I was so touched by the support from our friends and family that it brought me to tears. And each night, the meals arrived to sustain and nourish us, from our apartment building neighbors to our friends in Los Angeles. My sense of community and gratitude felt like it was taking over my whole body, one more weapon in my arsenal against the cancer.

Letters and packages arrived from all stages of my life, and even from people I didn't know. A stranger had heard my story—from whom I can't remember. But she sent me a thoughtful card and a care package with items to calm me during my treatment. I broke down as I read the heartfelt words from someone I had never even met.

And then there were my friends who showed up in so many different ways. Danielle jumped on a train from DC after my chemo infusions had begun. One of my closest friends from high school, she and I used to browse vintage clothing racks for the perfect 1970s-era polyester shirts, the funky-old-clothes mustiness thick in the air as we gabbed about everything. After college, we moved into our first apartment together, a roach-infested East Village studio that had been "converted" into a two bedroom. I was full swing into navigating my "What now?!" delayed adolescence, early-twenties freak-out. But our relationship survived that apartment and that freak-out. Years later, we traveled to Vietnam, stayed overnight in a houseboat in Halong Bay, and rode mopeds alongside rice paddies in the countryside. Danielle is one of those people who lives in my heart, always.

Lee, another cherished friend from high school, also dropped his responsibilities to spend the following weekend with me (he and Danielle had coordinated their visits). He was the first of my friends to hear about my potential diagnosis and knew just what to say to make me feel heard and loved.

Kat, my closest friend from college, flew all the way across the country from San Francisco to visit for the week and accompany me to treatment. Twenty-two years ago, our worlds collided when our college had run out of student housing and resorted to adding trailers to the campus. We were low in the housing lottery and ended up getting placed in a trailer together. Kat tolerated living with me when I was obsessed with George Michael's song "Freedom '90," which I played (loudly) on repeat for more than a few weeks. Kat is a woman of patience, passion, and adventure, and became someone so dear to me that I think of her as a sister.

Grateful was not an emotion that I anticipated feeling when I was diagnosed with cancer. And yet I felt it all the time. It often transcended my feelings of fear and anger. I became deeply aware of how wonderful my life was, how the people in it are outstanding and good, and that I am so lucky to be surrounded by my friends, family, my husband, and my girls. I wanted to hold on to my life with an unbreakable grip, but I knew I could lose it despite my desperation to stay alive.

Having a newborn can be an isolating experience. Fighting a life-threatening, physically debilitating, and energy-tapping illness can be an isolating experience. But I felt far from alone— I was cloaked in the warmth of my supportive community. It was incredibly moving.

At times, I found myself perplexed by all of the affection and care. Asking for help hasn't been one of my greatest strengths, largely because I worry about burdening others. Over the years, I have tried to work through those distorted thinking patterns in my own therapy, and to challenge myself by making requests. I've learned that people generally enjoy being helpful if given the chance. Nevertheless, there was a small part of me that wondered: if my friend visited from out of town, surely there was some other event that she needed to go to, and I was a pit stop on the way to the real destination. It seemed almost presumptuous to assume that people would show up for me in such a real and meaningful way.

But the evidence was right in front of me. My friends *wanted* to help me and I could count on them 100 percent. According to Bessel van der Kolk, relying on others in the aftermath of a traumatic event is "critical" to recovery; and in fact, the expression of emotion within one's support network is associated with longer survival for women with breast cancer.[1, 2] I needed to be cared for, and my vulnerability was teaching me the invaluable lesson that it's OK to ask for help, that I don't need to do everything on my own.

My friends cried with me. One girlfriend offered to meet me in Central Park so that we could scream at the top of our lungs. They didn't shy away from talking about my fear of dying, of abandoning my girls. They stayed steady with me and held me, literally, through my emotional and physical pain. I felt their love, and it felt so good. Though it was certainly a disaster, cancer had opened my eyes to the profound significance of my beloved relationships.

28

A TWISTED SPINE

It was a typical nonworkday in the summer of 2018: wake up to say good morning to the girls; morning nap; physical therapy; then massage therapy; work phone calls; taking the girls to the dentist. The dental appointment finished up earlier than I had anticipated, and I had time to make it to a slow-flow yoga class I had recently started attending—an hour of gentle stretches which had been approved by my physical therapy team.

I felt stiff, tight, and unsteady. The poses that were once second nature to me were literally out of reach. I tired easily and spent much of the class curled up on my mat in the restorative "child's pose." But little by little, week by week, I was surprised that I was starting to feel stronger and more limber. I focused on taking deep breaths in and out of my increasingly able body.

Then one day, within the series of lying-on-the-mat yoga instructions the teacher said, "And twist your spine . . ." My eyes were closed but immediately welled up, tears flowing alongside my temples and forming little saltwater pools in my ears. I remembered the doctors' words that I would never be able to twist my spine again without risk of fracture. I remembered what I used to feel only eight months before: the pain, immobility, and betrayal. I remembered the time when my body would not cooperate with my demands, even taking a step or two. Yet there I was, lying on my back and carefully moving my bent knees like windshield wipers from one side of my body to the other. I felt the stretch in my lower back and along the length of my torso. There was a healthy feeling of release and openness.

Somatic-based approaches to trauma recovery highlight the importance of providing patients with physical experiences that confront the physical immobilization and helplessness associated with the trauma. Unlike traditional talk therapy, where meaning-making often takes the form of a narrative, in somatic-focused therapies engaging the body is considered essential in healing from trauma.[1] Standard verbal-oriented talk therapy may miss the opportunity to uncover and process traumatic memories that were not encoded as explicit declarative memories, which you might be able to string into a narrative and make meaning out of, but as implicit sensory traces or fragments with no storyline.[2]

In *Sensorimotor* and *Somatic Experiencing* therapies, for example, the inability to escape one's terrifying circumstances is considered to be the driver of trauma-related symptoms; therefore, the opposite behavior—the body generating fight-or-flight-like movements—is believed to counteract the internalization of the body and self as powerless.[3, 4] Therapy focuses on increasing perceptual awareness of subtle internal body sensations, also known as *interoception*, and engaging in empowered actions, referred to as "acts of triumph," that were impossible during the traumatic incident.[5] Patients are also encouraged to use their bodies to "discharge" the buildup of fight-flight-freeze energy by allowing themselves to "shake," which according to Somatic Experiencing founder Peter Levine is a natural and essential body response that must be released after being traumatically paralyzed.[6]

In somatic-focused psychotherapies, trauma memories are elicited and the body is encouraged to move in ways that provide a corrective experience. This challenges the previous mind-body experience of being a helpless trauma victim; the felt sense of the body is grounded and strong, resulting in cognitive and emotional changes and restoring a much-desired sense of control. An example of a somatic-focused therapeutic technique is abruptly lifting and tensing the arms and hands to indicate *STOP!* in a gesture of self-defense.[7] For survivors of assault, patients may even take self-defense classes to encourage this type of movement. Not surprisingly, somatic therapists also often recommend yoga.[8] Combining mindfulness meditation, physical postures, and a focus on the breath, yoga is research-supported as an adjunctive treatment for trauma (and diabetes, insomnia, asthma—the list continues). One study found that weekly one-hour yoga classes over a ten-week period significantly reduced chronic posttraumatic stress disorder symptoms in women who had been "treatment-resistant," or nonresponsive, to psychotherapy or medication.[9] Results suggested that the interoceptive-building and physical aspects of yoga were likely responsible for traumatic symptom relief.

During this stage of trauma recovery, a new relationship emerges between the self and body in which the latter is (tentatively) trusted once again. The betrayal of the earlier trauma recovery days begins to fade. In my case, during those first few months of beginning my yoga practice again, I cried in or

throughout the majority of the classes. They were tears of sadness, fear, hope, mourning, and gratitude. It was a strange shift
in my emotional state, for sure, as I had wondered, back in
those days of fighting for my life, if I would ever find my tears
and be awakened from the numbness that had become my new
reality.

Physical activity, and yoga in particular, unfurled my emotions until they poured out of me in a therapeutic release. I
sobbed as I moved in ways I never thought would be possible,
twisting my spine and touching my toes with ease. The cognitions I had held on to as truths, that my body would forever be
unable to engage in certain positions because of the risk of fracture, turned out to be false. This shift in thinking and knowing
opened what felt like a whole world of possibility.

Though my body holds the memory of being held captive
by a deadly force, that force was finally quieted—I could move
again.

29

MANCALA

There will always be a part of me that appreciates Liz Phair and her rebellious contemporaries. Though after several months, the cancer-induced adolescent-like angst started to melt away.

It was as if I were viewing the world through a new set of eyes. There was a ripeness to experience. Everything looked different from even the precancer life that I had lived. Now each step, my foot against the pavement, felt like a miracle. The warm, golden sunshine on my face and the act of squinting my eyes to shield them from the glare, felt like gifts. I was ALIVE. Only a few months prior, I had prepared myself for a whole lot of lasts; now my life had become a new set of firsts.

I was at the beginning stages of rebuilding the other parts of my identity that I so valued: I was an engaged parent, back at work, and a romantic and present partner with my husband. But this transformation from unable to able didn't happen all at once. I had my good days and my not-so-good days. The immunotherapies continued to cause significant fatigue, skin reactions, headaches, and nausea and thus inhibited my ability to be the consistently adventurous, active family member that I had been previously.

Many of my waking hours were still spent tending to my cancer-patient status. Every morning and night I would open my two-gallon ziplock bag filled with an impressive array of medications and supplements. I hoped, as I swallowed them down, that they would support my body in its continual fight against the cancer. In addition to the cancer-related pills, I also took Lexapro (an antidepressant) and Ativan (an antianxiety), as I had since I had become a mom five years prior.

After I gave birth to Sophie, I was plagued with anxiety, guilt, and self-doubt. I was certain that my thoughts and feelings were proof that I was a bad mom. I was *shoulding* all over myself, judging my emotional state because *wasn't I supposed to be in maternal bliss?* I had always dreamed of becoming a mother, but once I did, I felt betrayed and disgusted by what I viewed as my inherent lack of maternal instincts. My internal dialogue repeated the same cruel phrases: *You're not cut out for this. You're failing as a mother.* I was in therapy, but the stickiness of my self-loathing cognitions required an additional intervention, and so I began taking an antidepressant.

Within weeks, my self-judgments, hopelessness, and anxiety dissipated. I, like so many other parents who suffer from postpartum anxiety or depression, had misconstrued my symptoms as a window into my "true" personality. But when they were no longer front and center, I could clearly see that I was not my symptoms, and, in fact, I was a good mom. It is with much relief that I can write that I have not suffered from postpartum depression or anxiety since I began taking psychiatric medication to treat the condition.

Then one morning, postcancer, I woke up (sort of) after a fit-

ful night's sleep. That old, familiar visitor was with me. I struggled to get myself out of bed, let alone outside. Once outdoors,
all I saw was the grayness of the sky. It was as if I could feel
the oppressive overcast descending upon me. I felt a simulta-
neous concoction of joylessness, emptiness, and anger. I was
depressed.

I noticed a woman walking toward me with long blond hair.
Then I saw another with long brown hair. And standing on the
sidewalk was a gorgeous woman with straight, silky hair pulled
back into a ponytail, her hair reaching midway down her back.
All of these women looked so elegant, feminine, and healthy.
How had I not noticed them fully before? Beautiful women
were everywhere! And I certainly wasn't one of them.

I was pissed. I wanted my hair and its original color back. I
thought to myself, My skin is breaking out from the immunotherapy treatments. I am sickly pale. My hair (what little I have
of it) is a dull brown. My body is still misshapen. And I am so
incredibly exhausted.

I knew that I was viewing the world through a negative lens.
It was as if I had left my clear glasses at home. Despite knowing
that my thoughts were depression-induced, my anger was real
and I didn't know where to put it. I went to bed that night in fear
that the darkness had taken its hold and would be with me for
who-knows-how-long.

The next day, thankfully, I woke up feeling like myself again.
I wasn't weighted down by my heavy eyelids, which had been
at half-mast the day before. It was gray outside again because it
was a rainy day, not because I was depressed.

I tried to piece together what had happened over the previous forty-eight hours that could have triggered such an abrupt
and intense shift in mood. There had been no situational

trigger. I had taken my Lexapro (an antidepressant) each night, as I had ever since I had become a mom five years ago. But as I thought back to my bag of pill bottles, I realized that I had mistakenly taken a lower dose of Ativan (an antianxiety)—and that was likely the culprit in setting off my depression and severe exhaustion. I was in benzodiazepine withdrawal (which is nothing to sneeze at)! Years ago during my doctoral training, I had provided psychotherapy at an inpatient unit where patients with benzodiazepine addiction were slowly tapered off the drugs in order to avoid potential dangerous withdrawal effects, including seizures. My broken sleep, depression, irritability, and exhaustion were all textbook symptoms of Ativan withdrawal.

That pill bag was just too big and unwieldy, and the possibility of inadvertently skipping over one bottle was clearly too high. I needed to simplify my medication routine and reduce the likelihood of a missed dose.

So I bought myself a weekly medication organizer with morning and evening compartments. It's become a little ritual now; once a week I sit cross-legged on my bed with all of my pill bottles and, one by one, I open the bottles, take out the pills, and drop them into their rightful A.M. and/or P.M. containers.

The sound of each pill landing in the case—*kuplink, kuplink, kuplink*—transports me back to the age of seven when I would play my favorite childhood game, Mancala. I remember the sensation of the game's colorful, smooth gems in my hand and their satisfying sounds as they made contact with the wooden game board. And my delight when I was rewarded by landing in a big pile of gems. I got to pick each of them up, my little child hand feeling especially small as I tried to hold all of the pieces and add them to my keep.

Now I carefully check to make sure that the correct pill doses land in their proper compartments. Sometimes I wonder, How much of my relative steadiness during this cancer ordeal has been because of them? It's certainly not something I plan to test out beyond that one-day accidental experiment.

30

HISTORY CAN'T GUIDE US

The morning of our wedding, back in August 2010, Derek and I woke up together in our hotel bedroom, excited for the day ahead. Derek was planning on showering, shaving, and donning his suit at the bed-and-breakfast where his family was staying. I had the makeup artist and hairstylist arriving at my parents' house at 9:00 A.M. I was on a tight schedule, with final wedding decisions to make before meeting with the venue organizer and photographer later that morning. There was much to do on that momentous day!

After brushing our teeth and putting on our nonwedding, casual attire, Derek asked that we sit at the bar at the hotel's restaurant and order lattes before going off on our separate, getting-ready-for-the-wedding adventures. It was a sweet idea, but I told him no, we will need to get the coffees to go. I had to get to my parents' house in time for my preparations.

And thus commenced one of the biggest, most dramatic, and perhaps the stupidest fight we have ever had. Derek was completely thrown by my lack of flexibility (which he reminded me is a repeat offense on my part—he may be right), my insistence upon him driving me to my parents' house to get ready *now*. I was astounded by his hot demand to add yet another activity to my already bloated list of to-dos; clearly, I wouldn't be able to enjoy even a half-sip of latte at that bar.

We didn't get the coffees to go. I remember sitting beside Derek in the front seat of the car, seething in silent anger. He unceremoniously dropped me off, no kisses or I-love-yous as we parted, and then went on his way, presumably buying a coffee somewhere without me. I set up camp in my parents' tiny bathroom and wept.

How could I marry a guy who was *so* insensitive to my needs? Why would he blow up today, *of all days*, over a latte? My mother knocked on the bathroom door and then entered the cramped space, interrupting my wedding day breakdown. She stood above me, a clump on the cool tile floor, and said calmly, "Just marry him today, honey. You can always divorce him next week."

So I got ready: makeup applied, the fragrant gardenia pinned into my hair, and my white lace wedding dress slipped on. Derek and I met at the ceremony site with the photographer for the "first look" pictures. When we saw each other, we burst into tears of love and, I think, relief.

In retrospect, I realize that we were grappling with a heavy helping of prewedding jitters. But still, a fight of that magnitude, over a fucking latte?

Oh, the joys of relationships. Derek and I have been at it for twenty years now, no strangers to conflict, to missing each other's cues, to driving each other up the wall. We have our go-to arguments, the same themes emerging time and time again. How we manage time, as evidenced in the wedding morning snafu, is a consistent one. I want to leave for the airport early in case of unforeseen traffic, long lines at security, or one of our children having a blowout poop episode (this shit scenario actually happened on one occasion and we barely made our flight). Derek would like to leave without any padding, because for him, extra time spent at the airport is a waste of what could be much better spent at home or on vacation.

You'd think that we would have figured out how to navigate this issue long ago, but it took years—years!—before we identified our individual travel wants, communicated them clearly, and then collaborated and agreed upon a plan that made us both feel supported and relatively anxiety-free.

Cleanliness is another point of division. I play the "what has Derek been up to today" game around our apartment, following his tracks. The pantry cabinet door is open, cookie crumbs on the floor. Seeds are sprinkled on the counter near the toaster beside a stray piece of that waxed paper insert that separates the slices of our packaged Muenster cheese. Derek obviously toasted a piece of our seeded multigrain bread and made a melted cheese sandwich. And at some point, helped himself to a cookie . . . or two . . . There's a coffee cup on the dining table. On our side table next to the couch is a bowl with a spoon resting in it, remnants of milk at the bottom, likely left out overnight: evidence of his late-night cereal habit. Derek is oblivious to the fact that he has left a traceable trail. But I encounter every object as glaringly-out-of-place.

When I was five months pregnant with Sophie, Derek and I lived on the sixth floor of a walk-up in Chelsea. It was not family-friendly—neighbors smoked cigarettes in the hallways, raucous parties echoed through the paper-thin ceilings and walls until the wee hours of the night, and hordes of visitors ran up and down the stairs to access the roof to do God knows what. So it was with surprise that Derek returned home from his graduate school classes one evening to find that I had left my keys to the apartment still in the keyhole outside our door. He said to me, with loving concern, that it was not safe to leave my keys in the door like that. I was shocked that I had left them there to begin with, and told him so.

But then the next day Derek returned home and he was greeted by those same keys, dangling from the keyhole, *again*. I couldn't believe it—but the proof was in Derek's hand. I blamed my back-to-back absentmindedness on "pregnancy brain." But I also learned an important lesson.

It took me a long while to recognize that Derek's messiness is not purposeful; he simply doesn't realize that he leaves his stuff everywhere. He doesn't *see* it. And so I try my best to remember the key scenario when I feel like I'm reaching my boiling point from picking up after my husband from kitchen to dining area to couch to bedroom. My remembering helps me to more calmly remind Derek that it makes me feel less anxious and more at peace in our home when it looks tidy.

The theme of presence is another biggie in our relationship. Derek is an extraordinary thinker—he gets lost in his thoughts and sometimes will walk a few paces ahead of me, not realizing it, because he is so deep in his own world. I see the back of him, but want him by my side. I used to interpret this drifting as an indication of his lack of interest in me. But over the years (and much therapy), I have learned that Derek's forging ahead is an aspect of his personality that has zero to do with me. And that insight takes the hurt out.

Derek is a workhorse. His dedication to his job is unlike any I've ever seen. He is a partner at a major consulting group where he pours all of himself into his projects and teams, always searching for the best answers to questions that I will simply never, ever, understand. Under no circumstance could I come close to comprehending the work he does, and he in turn has told me that he could never fathom the work of a psychologist. So how is it that two such different brains fell in love? Is it our differences that brought us together?

Sometimes, Derek is so engrossed in his work that he can't hear me or see me because of his focus on the task at hand. I'm like that coffee mug he's left on the dining room table; there, but not there. It does provide me with reassurance to know that Derek's behaviors are not specific to me. His colleagues nicknamed him "Neo" after Keanu Reeves's character in *The Matrix* because of his unusual ability to be plugged into work despite conversations happening all around him. Me, ever the psychologist—I yearn for his eye contact and validation, reflecting back what I've shared with him. But that's not always what I get. And I know that I chose Derek partly for that reason. He's driven and independent, like me. I get the space that I need to pursue my interests. But also, I think that I was drawn to Derek because he's a *challenge*.

When he is fully present with me (computer and cell phone out of reach), there comes a big payoff, the warmth of his beautiful eyes resting on me alone. It's slightly unsettling when I admit to myself the truth of the matter—that I think I would be bored with an always available, always sympathetic, and always emotionally available partner. What does that say about me?

Like many other couples, Derek and I have different relationship barometers. He is typically pretty content in our relationship no matter what, and when asked will likely report we're at 100 percent, doing great. But sometimes I think his measuring device is off-kilter. I believe that there is room for improvement, work to be done, a greater connection that can be sowed. So, with a not-so-subtle nudge from me, we talk about our wants and how to better manage them together. And often through a combination of acceptance and compromise, we find the solutions.

This isn't really a fair assessment of our relationship tiffs because you're reading only my side of the story. I'm sure Derek would have no problem filling pages with tales about my relational blind spots and challenging behaviors. I imagine that inflexibility, demandingness, and emotional intensity may be my top three offenses. We come together with our own histories, our own baggage, our own worldviews that may be strikingly at odds at times. But after all these years, and all of our countless arguments, we are here, together still.

You never know how someone will respond to a significant trauma, like witnessing your pregnant wife literally fall apart, cancer eating her alive until she'll likely be dead. Derek floored me in his steadiness, his compassion, his devotion to me and our family. Like me, he had operated in full-speed-ahead mode at the height of the crisis. He was rock solid, present with me at that 100 percent mark right beside me for five straight months of cancer-induced hell, and made me feel more love than ever in my entire life.

The hard part came after the tornado had dissipated and we had to pick up the remaining pieces of ourselves, but felt as if there was no foundation on which to settle in this new, sort-of-postcancer reality. Derek had lost most of me from the September 2017 diagnosis until February of the next year, unable to get around without a walker, and stricken with significant side effects from chemo and immunotherapy. When I was declared NED, we knew that I had become one of the luckiest ones, who had fared, thus far, better than 94 percent of women with my same diagnosis.[1] We didn't know what recovery would look like, but in the meantime, I was nowhere near the partner Derek had had before the cancer diagnosis.

The meal train that my friend set up was such a gift, but one day it stopped. Like when sitting shiva—the Jewish tradition of supporting mourners—comes to an end, life goes on, but not in the same way. Derek was back at work. We had less support. We were fragmented and worn down. It was clear that I had just undergone a huge trauma, but Derek had, too. It wasn't until the dust had settled, somewhat, that he was able to fully reckon with the fear, anger, loss, disappointment, and pretty much every other emotion there is out there.

Support networks, including family members, may have all hands on deck as cancer patients undergo chemotherapy, but they are often less prepared for what can be a slow, and at times seemingly stagnant, rate of recovery in the treatment's aftermath.[2] This was very much the case in our family, as after the crisis had subsided, I was nowhere near back to my previous level of functioning. It's not surprising that frustration is a common response among partners who are confronted with the reality that their loved ones are not their previous selves and continue to be incapable of keeping up with ordinary day-to-day events.[3]

Derek's trauma reaction, which included the frustration noted above or a complete emotional shutdown, was consistently triggered in our new norm of daily living. One weekend I would build up his sense of hope, he witnessing me being able to spend hours with him and the girls, and then the next weekend I'd be in bed, wiped. I had learned quickly that if I said *Yes* when I knew that my body wanted me to say *No*, that I would pay royally for overexerting myself. But it was still so hard to say no. Derek would make weekend plans with friends for us, and I would routinely bow out from exhaustion. Each time I canceled it seemed like a stab to his heart. Another letdown, Derek yet again the stag parent, the taker of both kids to Sophie's classmate's birthday party, while his wife was in bed at home, sleeping. He wanted me back as his wife, his all-around partner. But my status was so touch-and-go that Derek couldn't rely on me.

To make matters all the more confusing, there was no specific endpoint that we were working toward or could look forward to. I had already reached the best-case scenario of NED. But our life was far from rainbows and sunshine. No one could tell us if the cancer would reinvade my body, or how soon that day would come. How do you recover from a trauma that is an ongoing part of one's daily life?

Derek was like a ghost version of his former self, his body like a shell containing all of his hurt. He had started his own personal therapy but had difficulty connecting with a clinician. He retreated into his own trauma world—distant, no warm and fuzzies. And after those five months of absolutely no conflict whatsoever, we started to argue.

Just weeks before my cancer diagnosis, Derek, Sophie, and I had had professional maternity photos taken, with the plan for newborn sessions two months later, when our new family member arrived. I remember the photographer asking me to lie down on the grass, and my telling her that I couldn't get in that position because of my hip pain. None of us knew it at the time, but that pain was because of the large tumor feasting on my bones. After the diagnosis, not surprisingly, that newborn photo shoot never actualized.

When I was starting to recover from chemo, I asked Derek, Should we do that photo shoot now? Delayed, but at least when Siena was still an infant?

Derek replied, "Are you sure you want to do the photo shoot with your hair like that?"

I felt my eyes and brow tighten, the anger rising to the surface with my zinger of a reply, "Well, we could wait longer, but then there's the risk I could be dead by then."

I would *not* label this a healthy moment of communication. His words stung, and I upped the ante, stinging him right back. But in retrospect, I can also understand that my physical appearance in itself was a trauma trigger for Derek. I looked sick. Why would he want professional photographs of one of his biggest trauma triggers—his sick wife—hanging around his apartment and sent around to family and friends?

I couldn't accelerate my healing or the growth of my buzzed-short hair and felt powerless to improve things between us. We were both so raw, fumbling in the dark, not knowing how to be together. Our interactions didn't look pretty; our words weren't always the kindest or most loving. We are human, after all, and were slogging through how to emerge from the scariest time in our lives.

Our arguments were all the more complicated because they were different from our standard fights. There were no relationship themes to fall back on. In the past, we could recognize and quickly rectify our spats by reenacting the familiar solutions that sometimes fell to the wayside and needed resurrecting. But these new arguments were uncharted territory. We had no playbook to turn to, no history to guide us.

I often tell my patients that arguing is a skill. If enacted effectively, communicating about the most difficult aspects of one's relationship can help propel it forward, engendering necessary change to meet new relational demands. But Derek and I were rendered skill-less by the cancer, like two boxers in a ring stripped of their protective gear. No helmets, no gloves, and certainly no referee.

On the bright side, it was safe again to argue. There had been no space for us to fight during the crisis months because we were at a standstill. Life had been whittled down to the singular goal of trying to keep me alive, and we were on the same page there. But now I *was* alive, which opened the potential for expectations, yearnings, and (many) disappointments.

Derek and I needed to relearn how to argue skillfully, to figure out how to negotiate the new set of facts that were our life. In our traumatized states, this was no easy task. I think Derek described this time in our lives perfectly: our relationship was not a light switch you could just turn on again; we were at a low dim for a long time. But with hard work in couples therapy and our continued dedication to our relationship, we learned how to love each other all over again.

31

TABLE 5

One of my friends from high school invited Derek and me to celebrate his marriage. David and I had spent much of our formative years together—on his back patio on the Upper West Side, in Central Park, or listening to live music at Smalls in Greenwich Village. David introduced me to jazz and blues, and he was the friend I called whenever I was stumped on a crossword puzzle answer and needed to borrow a brain. Like when I called David to ask him the seven-letter word for a portable grill, he answered immediately: "Hibachi."

I was excited about David's wedding, his finding love. It was also fun to think about seeing our high school "guy crew" there, some of whom I had lost touch with over the years. But I was a cancer patient now. I looked different and felt different. What would it be like to go to a party? I hadn't been at a multihour evening gathering for over a year.

This was a huge postcancer-diagnosis leap, so unfamiliar after being bed-bound, in a dissociative fog, and then further cut off from "outside of myself" experiences like socializing, because

TABLE 5   165

of my brain's insistence on ruminating about my cancer status only. I was nervous, and the anxiety-laden thoughts started to mount: Would I tire and need to go home early? Would anyone ask about my cancer? Do I bring it up during the inevitable "so, what have you been doing with your life for the last XX years" conversation? My answer to that question was only hinted at by my short hair. But I wondered, for those who were meeting me for the first time—did my hair look like a style, and not a sickness?

At this stage of trauma recovery, there is a reengagement with the self and the building of a new identity; at first, this translated to me feeling like a stranger to myself and a foreigner in my own life. For many trauma survivors, the nascent stages of rebuilding the sense of self often results in an isolated, inner-focused life experience, and relationships become a source of confusion.[1] Trauma can also damage self-esteem and result in feeling awkward and uncertain about how to interact with people effectively. I took my insecurities with me to the wedding, worrying, wondering, and feeling unsure about how to present myself.

When we arrived at the event, it was raining, so we guests huddled together, shielding ourselves on David's family's back porch under umbrellas. It felt cozy and celebratory. Soon the sky cleared and Derek and I found our seating card and made our way to Table 5. I sat next to Sean, another friend from high school whom I hadn't seen in years. The rest of those at the table were unknown to me at the beginning of the night, but I quickly felt at ease with each of them, and soon my belly ached from boisterous laughter.

My tablemates discussed aging, back pain, and physical therapy. The presumed invincibility of our teens and early twenties had been replaced with the group admission that our bodies are in fact fallible (though there was humor to these late-thirtysomethings complaining like eighty-year-olds). Yes, I could certainly contribute to that conversation. But I remained mute and simply listened.

I was the psychologist from Manhattan. The mom of two girls. But it was at the tip of my tongue: *I've also been in physical therapy! I couldn't walk! Today I walked three miles!* But is it appropriate to talk about the big C at Table 5? Will it lead to awkward silences, the flow and levity in conversation forever altered? When and how do I share this significant, almost all-consuming part of myself? How can I be authentic, open, and contribute to the discussion without scaring off my tablemates? Will people want to hang out with the cancer girl at the party?

I imagined that saying aloud "I have cancer" would have been the equivalent to me jumping up and down, exclaiming, "Hey, y'all want to talk about death and dying?!" That's a far cry from the wedding table chitchat I've had in my day. You don't talk about trauma at a wedding. Everyone knows that. It's a party, there's free booze flowing, and the objective is a good time to be had by all. So I decided that "cancer Sarah" would be on vacation that night, and I had a great time.

I think I came across as healthy and very much alive.

32

LIVING IN IT

There's a lot of time spent indoors when you're fighting cancer. For many months, my view of the world was mostly limited to the four walls of my bedroom as I contemplated Virginia Woolf's description of the healthy "army of the upright" continuing their "marches to battle" on the New York City streets below.[1] Thankfully, I lived on a high floor of an apartment building, which provided me with a view of the cityscape facing south. As grateful as I was for that window, I yearned to see something green. A tree, some grass, a flower. I missed the fresh country air and the comfort and calm that nature brings. With the holidays upon us, Derek, the romantic that he is, was trying to come up with a meaningful present for me. He knew what I wanted most was access to nature, but being ill and confined to bed made that fantasy unattainable.

We tried purchasing a small evergreen tree for our family. In less than a week, we had managed to kill it; the needles turned brown and branches drooped, sadly, toward the floor.

So Derek thought way outside the box and decided to bring

the outdoors in to me—and in a way that wouldn't remind us even more of our mortality. Derek bought me a painting of an Italian country landscape and hung it opposite our bed. Vineyards and cypress trees filled the background, and in the foreground were lush trees, heavy with all shades of green leaves. Tied to the branches of two trees was a line, and hanging from that line were clothes, drying in the Tuscan sun. There was what looked like a bedsheet, pants, blouses—and smaller leggings that must have belonged to a child. The shaded, undulating lines in the grass and position of the hanging clothes gave away that it had been a windy day when the painter was at his easel. Looking at that painting, it seemed as if I could feel the breeze and smell the fresh air, even though I was apartment-bound in New York City.

I spent hours staring into that painting. It always changed, depending on the time of day and the way the light filtered in through our window. I got lost in it and felt transported from my four-wall-world to a place of expansiveness and serenity.

It's not always possible for cancer patients to take a vacation. If you are able to, the change of scenery can be incredibly healing. Maybe that means having someone drive you just an hour away from home to a wooded area or a lake. Gift your brain and senses with that different view and place. But please, if you travel abroad, heed my humble advice: don't go to any country with questionable drinking water.

Derek and I learned this the hard way when we took an "I'm done with chemo" celebratory trip, two months post my last dose, to just north of Puerto Vallarta, Mexico. In my chemotherapy-suppressed immune system state, I immediately acquired traveler's diarrhea and spent the three-day vacation on the toilet, not the beach.

Luckily, this was not our only trip planned for the year. After we learned that I was NED, my parents announced to me, Derek, my brother, and his family that we were going to Italy! Six months after my NED designation, all ten of us piled into an Italian home situated next to rolling vineyards and hues of green as far as the eye could see. When we arrived, my father, brother, and I walked barefoot through the backyard. The textures of the grass and twigs felt like a massage under my naked, city-girl feet. The three of us stood in silence and looked out at the majesty before us. Mother nature got it right in Italy. Standing there, feeling the breeze against my skin, seeing the cypresses jutting out of the land like in a Van Gogh, I realized—I was *in* the painting that Derek had bought for me.

Throughout that trip, it was as if someone had turned up the volume and I was hearing, seeing, and tasting for the first time in almost a year. Bites of pasta felt like bursts of savory flavors on my previously chemo-induced, metallic-tasting-only tongue. The way the sunlight landed, it seemed to be caressing everything it touched. Hearing the familiar yet foreign sounds of the Italian language roused a part of my brain that I hadn't realize had been asleep. I discovered that there is a much bigger world out there than my cancer-fighting bedroom.

33

A NEW TREATMENT PLAN

I had an incredible summer. Italy had awakened my illness- and trauma-dulled senses. I came home from the trip with my eyes fully open to the world around me, and I was excited to be an active participant in it.

As I got further out from the chemotherapy treatments, there were moments when I almost started to feel like my precancer self again. Derek commented with a smile when he noticed that I had hung fresh eucalyptus in our shower; I was starting to tend to the small details of our lives, with joy, and was feeling creative energy again.

Though by the end of that summer in 2018, seemingly out of nowhere, my body felt as if it had abruptly shut down. At first, I accepted the rapid decline as a reality of continuing cancer immunotherapy infusions. I assumed that the symptoms were temporary and would resolve on their own. But after months of feeling weak, dizzy, and zombie-like, I sat in Dr. Dang's office and cried.

My treatment plan, for life, was to receive Herceptin and

Perjeta infusions every three weeks. After only a year of accumulating treatments, however, my body had entered a state of collapse. Once again, the fatigue took over. I slept in late in the mornings and took afternoon naps. I was able to get through my two workdays each week but needed a day or two in bed thereafter to recuperate. I felt as if I were moving through mud. My skin was covered in a spotted rash that itched like mad and often woke me in the middle of the night. I took frequent rounds of antibiotics in an attempt to treat the infection that ravaged my skin, blanketing it with severe acne. Countless pink mounds protruded from every square inch of my face; the antibiotics were no match for the cancer medications' side effects. My blood pressure, historically always in the low range, was now even lower, hovering around 90/45. I found it difficult to move around, always light-headed and exhausted. Thrust back into the role of an ill cancer patient, I wondered, Was *this*—not the Italian-vista version of my life—my new normal?

According to my doctor, the significant side effects were likely being caused by the Perjeta. Researchers aren't certain how long Perjeta remains in one's system, but it was clear that I was "saturated" with the immunotherapy and had reached my max. Without hesitating, Dr. Dang told me that we would stop the Perjeta for now to give my body a break, and see if the pause would reduce some of the distressing side effects.

Altering the treatment plan was both a significant relief and absolutely terrifying. We knew that the combination of Perjeta and Herceptin had killed the cancer cells in my body quickly and efficiently. How much of my response was because of the Perjeta? If I took a break from Perjeta, would the cancer immediately awaken from its previous dormant state?

As a psychologist, I was familiar with the concept of testing hypotheses—but this seemed to be a pretty risky experiment.

Dr. Dang assured me that Herceptin is the main immuno-therapy agent used to fight Her2 positive breast cancer, and that for many years, it was the only immunotherapy available to combat the disease. Perjeta is the adjunct to Herceptin, the extra helper that can boost Herceptin's effectiveness. Dr. Dang explained that my sensitivity to the drugs (super-responder status!) also likely resulted in super side effects—and she believed that it was worth the risk to take me off Perjeta to see if I could live a more comfortable and able life. She reminded me of the "art" to our treatment plan, as there is limited data on NED metastatic breast cancer patients. We would continue to monitor me closely: evaluating my cancer blood levels every three weeks and regular PET/CT scans to check for visible tumors.

Within two months after stopping the Perjeta, my blood pressure returned to 90/60, which was the normal range for me. My skin itching and acne-form facial rashes were finally largely responsive to medication. Gradually, the faintness lifted and my energy improved. I didn't always need a morning nap. And some days I went without any nap at all.

I was feeling better physically, but my emotional functioning started to falter. I was back in that uncomfortable world of uncertainty-induced anxiety again. We had changed a major variable in my treatment—and none of us knew what the implications would be. Was the choice to live with debilitating side effects, or to die?

As the date for my PET/CT scan grew nearer, I found myself in a state of panic. I attributed every bodily sensation to the likelihood that the cancer had relodged itself in my body, the Perjeta no longer at work to keep it at bay. For example, there was a bizarre tingling sensation that traveled from my right hip down to my foot; it felt as if warm water were running down my leg. I was convinced that a new tumor was sitting on a nerve in my pelvic area and was causing this unusual symptom. My hair and nails were brittle and tearing, as they had been when the cancer was at its peak. Surely, I thought, the disease was directing resources away from supporting my healthy cells in order to promote the proliferation of the cancer cells . . . etcetera . . . ad infinitum.

The PET/CT results came back clean. My family and I sobbed as we took in the news. We would proceed with Herceptin only, and hoped that I would continue to feel better the further out I got from the Perjeta treatments. Now I imagine Herceptin as my Spider-Man—so formidable that he does not need Robin or any other sidekick to maintain order in my body.

34

THE DRAGONFLY

Following my discharge from physical therapy after six months of hard work, the unthinkable happened: I was able to run. Moving swiftly through space, feeling the rush of air tickling my bare arms and face, aroused near ecstasy. I started slowly, knowing that my radiated pelvis was still finicky and could flare up with pain if I pushed myself too far or ran too fast.

Steadily, I increased my distance along the Hudson River in Riverside Park. Half a mile one day, maybe a full mile two days later. Listening to my body, I slowed to a walk when I tired.

Once I reached the two-mile mark, I felt a painful electric-like jolt in my right pelvic area with each running step, even when I reduced my speed. I spaced out my runs and reduced their mileage, hoping that I just needed a longer interval between sessions to let my muscles and ligaments recover. But each time I returned to running, the same pain resurfaced. Sometimes it became so persistent that I walked with a limp for a week after a gentle jog. Running provoked that radiated pelvic spot in a not-OK way.

Precancer, I had dreams of participating in 5Ks and maybe a half- or full marathon one day. So I sought out physical therapy again, hoping that with expert guidance, my body would relearn how to adjust to the activation of that persnickety pelvic spot. But during and after each session, I experienced those pangs and lost the ability to engage in any sort of exercise for days or weeks thereafter. My persistence typically pays off, but after months of the accruing evidence that running induced pain and stagnation, I decided, enough. I can let this dream go. Ultimately, I decided that being able to walk without pain was more important to me than those fantasy 5Ks.

Before running became off-limits, I was out of the city one weekend and jogged for fifteen minutes straight, which was a personal postcancer record. On my slow cool-down walk back along the country road, I spotted a dragonfly.

It was on its back, its wings resting against the pavement. Trying with all of its might to flip onto its legs, it feverishly flapped its wings, but to no avail. I gently touched the dragonfly with my foot, attempting to turn it over, right side up. After multiple nudges, and even successful flips, the dragonfly somehow wound up on its back again, flailing.

I wondered, Is it dying? Is there no hope to save its life?

I found a large dried-up leaf and bent down to the pavement, up close with the creature. Carefully gliding the leaf underneath its wings, I turned the dragonfly over and waited. I watched. I marveled at its beautiful wings of blue, green, and teal. Glistening, transparent, and sparkling.

"OK, babe, now it's up to you to fly," I said, standing up. As I walked away I wondered, would it be able to take flight?

I think of that dragonfly often. Like that dragonfly, I was not sure of my physical limitations. For a long while, it was a game of trial and error to find out which movements I could engage in safely while remaining pain-free. I tried to listen to my body as it alerted me that I had pushed too far. I tried to respect its limits.

Luckily, I have found that the elliptical, walking, and yoga are all safe endeavors. Yoga actually has the opposite effect of running; the more I stretch, the better I feel, especially in that pelvic area. I'm amazed that I'm now able to contort my body into shapes that were never accessible prior to my cancer diagnosis, with zero protests from that radiated spot.

I enjoy my leisurely strolls and especially the breezier days that provide the heavenly sensation of wind caressing my exposed flesh. I feel like those dogs who happily hang their heads out of car windows, their furry faces and ears pulled back by the force of moving swiftly through the air. Each time I feel the touch of the wind, I am reminded: I am alive.

Every week back in 2019, I took Siena to her toddler "forest class" in Central Park. We both eagerly anticipated our time in the city's natural world together. We explored the hidden trails deep in the Ramble and visited streams, ponds, and her favorite mini-waterfall. We picked up leaves, acorns, and sticks to make mud stew in tin pails. I helped Siena climb a boulder, and once she reached the top, I placed my hands firmly under her arms and around her little back, lifting her high into the air as she "jumped off," and then swooped her dramatically down to the ground. Then she laughed and cried, intoxicatingly, "Again!"

I can keep up with Siena in the woods, crouch down to the earth to play and look for worms, and then fly mini-kites with her in the open field. I can love her. I can do what matters.

35

THE NEW HAT

I sat in the backseat of the taxi on the way to work, my professional clothes in place, but emotionally I was far from put together. I was sick again. It had been a while since I'd felt the sensation of tears, the welling around the edges of my eyes, the urgency with which I raised fingers to blot the wetness before it spilled and painted mascara-black streaks down my cheeks. I noticed the cabdriver catching glimpses of me, empathically, in his rearview mirror.

The 2019 to 2020 winter had been full of upper respiratory infections—similar to the previous winter, come to think of it. I was sick of being sick, of denying my little girls their cuddles for fear of getting them ill, the canceled plans, the lack of physical activity. I felt pissed off at the cancer for putting me in the position of having to contend with viruses for months on end. In desperation, I texted my oncologist, wondering why I had been feeling so rotten, and if she had any answers for me. She wrote that Herceptin could be "delaying my recovery" from these various illnesses.

As the taxi drove through Midtown Manhattan and passed St. Patrick's Cathedral, I steadied myself. Moments away from my office, I took some deep breaths, paid my driver (an extra tip for his rearview-mirror-kindnesses), and marched along East Forty-Ninth Street. Sitting opposite my clients, I shared emotional prescriptions that I, myself, was in dire need of.

Herceptin, my literal lifesaver, causes what Dr. Dang calls "itises" (translation: inflammation). For supersensitive me it means that while on this drug my skin (rash), nose (runny), lungs (congested), teeth (cavities), and even urethra (urgency to pee) are in a persistent, baseline state of irritation. When I get sick with a virus, the above symptoms intensify, and my routine is dismantled. My sinuses feel like they are going to explode from the pressure, my lungs are tight even after nebulizer treatments, and my body is faint and weak. It feels as if there's a weighty web of mucus just below my epidermis that has lodged itself throughout my brain, face, and lungs. It's hard for me to extract thoughts through that sticky, phlegmy barrier.

The protective layer on the linings of my throat, nose, esophagus, lungs, and stomach is missing—and this is a barrier that helps to ward off infection. The crease points in my armpits, the crook of my elbows, and where the edges of clothing meet my flesh (top of jeans, the collar of a shirt) are pink and itchy, sometimes swollen, chafed, and sore. I imagine—if my skin's sensitivity is anything like what's going on for me internally, then *oh, my poor insides!* No wonder I'm so susceptible to infections.

Sometimes I can trace my illnesses back to the exact moment of transmission. A few months ago, Siena was struck with a stomach virus in the middle of the night. After I removed her from her vomit-covered crib, Derek bathed our toddler as I maneuvered a change of the crib mattress sheet (which, at any hour, seems more difficult than earning a doctoral degree). I snuggled Siena—her hair still damp and fragrant from her bath—back to sleep, and placed her upon her clean sleeping spot. I returned to my own bed, but within thirty minutes, Siena was up again with another round of puke, and when I reached for her midprojectile, vomit landed just on the edge of my lower lip. I felt that tiny speck as if it were searing a hole in my flesh. I've been hit! Within twenty-four hours, I was hugging the toilet.

And when Sophie got her last cold that season, I knew that I was done for when she released an impressive spray-can sneeze, saliva shooting visibly out of her mouth. A drop landed, wet and cool, in my eye. Hit again! And down I went.

As a parent, it's part of the job description to be knee-deep in shit, mucus, and vomit. All of my family members recover in a normal time frame—a few days, maybe a week or ten days at most. But for me, that same infection can keep me down for a month and a half.

A few months prior to my winter illnesses, I eyed an item for sale at my yoga studio, the proceeds of which were going to cancer research. It was a black trucker hat with the words FUCK CANCER in pink neon, front and center.

I *needed* that hat, I thought, and bought it immediately. But it went straight into my closet, the defiant phrase looking out at me each time I opened the closet door. I was too chicken to wear it.

One day, in the throes of yet another infection, I was rallying to untether myself from the bed and go outside. I needed to go to the bank and buy some restorative soup. Then I remembered—that hat! I took a deep breath and told myself, Sarah, you're wearing it today. It would be a perfect way for me to practice accepting my rage at the cancer—and would up the ante by putting it on display for the world to see. And then there was the notion of disclosing my invisible cancer status to all of those around me, to boldly unmute myself by splaying the word CANCER across my forehead.

In psychology, we refer to this type of experiment as an "exposure." Some of us experience anxiety or discomfort when confronted with nonthreatening stimuli. The psychological treatment entails engaging in the very behavior that gives rise to the discomfort or anxiety, and over time, lo and behold, the distress abates. For a person with a fear of spiders, exposure treatment would involve creating a "fear hierarchy ladder" listing the least to most feared interactions with spiders. The lowest rung on this ladder may include looking at a photograph of a spider, whereas the highest rung may involve actually holding a live spider in one's hand. As the individual habituates to each of these hierarchy tasks, these once potentially highly upsetting experiences are no longer interpreted as threatening. We can live our lives guided by our goals and values as opposed to fear.

Though I wasn't afraid of my anger, I certainly didn't welcome it with open arms. I had tried to rationalize it away and, by doing so, had made myself feel guilty for feeling angry to begin with. Not a helpful cycle, especially considering that anger is a healthy and adaptive human emotion.

But what would it feel like to wear my anger for all to see? I would effectively be walking around my neighborhood carrying an anger torch. I anticipated that there would be looks of surprise from my city dwellers as they read the words (including an expletive) across my cap. As I made my way outside I felt the anticipatory anxiety start to rise—tightness in my chest and shallow breathing—evidence that the exposure was clearly at work.

I had totally misjudged my audience. I could walk around Manhattan with an inflatable inner tube around my waist, a bonnet on my head, and clown shoes on my feet and nobody would bat an eye. We New Yorkers pride ourselves on having *already seen it all*. Even in the face of celebrities, we're unflappable. The hat was just another hat.

I wore the hat, and though it felt awkward at first, I quickly saw that nobody cared, and I stopped caring, too. So I'm angry at cancer. No big deal! A few minutes into my errands I almost forgot about the message written across the front panel in bold. I had one last stop, to get my treat of a decaf cappuccino, before returning home to bed. Heading up to the counter, I saw that my favorite barista, Cassandra, was on her day shift. She also has cancer and, upon seeing me, immediately exclaimed, "OH MY GOD I LOVE YOUR HAT!" Cassandra asked me how I was feeling, and I answered truthfully, that this day wasn't my favorite—hence the hat. She told me that she was having a hard week, too. The side effects from her treatments were getting her down. We both listened to and supported each other. Our talk bolstered me, made me feel greater self-compassion, and granted me even more permission to fully experience all of my normal emotions.

Though the hat didn't explicitly indicate that *I* had cancer, to me, wearing that word was a bold experiment in disclosure. Up to that moment, I had been perpetually sizing up social situations, internally grappling with the question, *to share or not to share*, which was both distracting and, at times, exhausting. The hat threw that disclosure guessing game out the window.

For now, that hat is back in my closet. But I'm glad that I wore that hat. It's OK for me to feel angry. It's OK for me to display it, to wear it for all to see. And I know that it's there—and I can wear it again, like armor, on the days when I need it most.

36

UPSIDE DOWN

When I had been teeming with cancer, I felt divorced from my body. My primal fear necessitated a dissociative "I'm not here" state. Everything felt like it had been stripped away by the cancer during those months of chemo, hospital stays, and being confined to the bed or walker. And after the NED designation, I wasn't sure what was left of me, if anything. I had mostly checked out of my relationship with my own self. Life had a one-note quality to it. Sounds were muted. Colors, dull. The trauma- and chemo-triggered dissociative state served to de-intensify the more extreme parts of my life, both the good and the bad. I needed that detachment in order to get through the days.

As the initial cancer crisis continued to march further into my past, the dissociative defense was no longer necessary or helpful. But like being in a lucid dream, I knew that I still wasn't fully awake, and I didn't know how to rouse myself from psychological dormancy. I felt a sense of restlessness, that I needed to shake things up to feel vibrant again. And then I realized—it was time to reestablish a passionate relationship with my *self*.

In couples therapy, psychologists often highlight the importance of making time for each other (date nights), healthy communication, and novelty. Relationships can be thrilling in their early stages—the newness—the discovery—and the lust. That initial period can give way over time to what can feel more mundane. One great intervention to revitalize a couple is to prescribe that they do something out of the norm together. Take a day trip somewhere you've both never been. Try a couples cooking or painting class. Mix things up! Couples can take the novelty approach one step further by engaging in arousal-increasing experiences with each other—perhaps riding a roller coaster at a carnival or even rock climbing. Was there a way for me to adapt this dyadic intervention to my relationship with myself? I wanted to feel a surge of excitement that had been lacking for some time.

I may have a little thrill junkie in me. Years ago, I gifted Derek a skydiving certificate for his birthday. The present turned out to be more for me than for him. He was terrified, whereas I found flying through the sky exhilarating. Though I promised to never jump out of an airplane again once I became a mother.

I investigated and found out that I wasn't the only cancer patient looking for adventure. There are two organizations, Send It and First Descents, which provide food, lodging, and lessons in outdoor extreme sports for young (forty years and younger) cancer patients. I put myself on the wait list for a rock climbing excursion in Colorado and a white water rapids kayaking trip in Montana. I realized that rock climbing and rafting would be akin to voluntary direct exposures, as I would be engaging in fear- and arousal-inducing activities. But unlike the fear associated with a cancer diagnosis and all that it entails, these nature-based challenges would build much needed confidence in my body and its ability to manage stressful, though invigorating, circumstances.

I had to practice patience because the trips were popular, so it would be months or perhaps a year before I would get off the wait list. In the meantime, I wondered, Was there anything else I could do to inject vitality into my life?

I took my first yoga class when I was in college. My brother practiced yoga and had been encouraging me to give it a go for myself. So I went to a beginner class at his favorite yoga studio. I had two takeaways from that class: (1) Listen—try not to move until the teacher tells you what to do next. You may think you know what the instructor's going to say, but you are probably wrong; and (2) I suck at yoga.

Every time the teacher said, "And now, exhale . . ." I would inhale. When she said, "And now, inhale . . ." I would exhale. It's not that I have a problem with following directions. I just couldn't figure out how to get my body to sync up with her instructions. I looked around the room at each blissed-out face. It appeared that no one else was struggling with my issue. I thought, This isn't relaxing! And I'm in a beginner's class. If I can't figure out this simple breathing stuff, then clearly I'm not meant to be a yogi.

But why were all these people so in love with yoga? I was curious enough to stick with it. Eventually, I found my breath and was (mostly) able to connect it with my movements. Though I viewed yoga as simply a form of exercise, providing me with defined benchmarks of "achievement" that I could strive toward in new poses. Meditation and increasing body- and self-awareness were not part of my movement aspirations. There was no ohm-ing at the end of classes.

Many years later, after I got the green light from my oncological physical therapist that yoga was no longer off-limits, I decided to give it a go again. This time, however, I approached yoga from a new perspective. In the years since my first yoga classes I had started my own mindfulness practice and had read studies on the many psychological benefits of yoga. After enduring my cancer diagnosis and its aftermath, I wondered if a moving meditation could help me in my physical and emotional recovery.

I knew that I needed to start slow. I spent many months in gentle restorative yoga classes, finding my breath, a deep sense of relaxation, and the release of tears that had been caged inside my body during all of those months of trauma numbness. Like therapy in motion, yoga helped me tenderly reacquaint myself with my body and mind.

Then one day after six months of restorative classes, I decided to shake up the routine and try something new. I saw that there was a Level Two Vinyasa class that afternoon, and I figured, What the hell? I'll give it a go.

As I set up my mat, I noticed that I was surrounded by students who looked like professional athletes. The teacher walked in, instructed us to stand at the front of our mats, and then led us through a series of postures that were enormously challenging—but oh my God—I was having *fun*! I was clearly sticking out like a (very sweaty) sore thumb, not able to keep up or move my body like the other acrobatic yogis who were jumping effortlessly into gravity-defying positions, but I had a

smile plastered across my flushed face for the whole class. My
body was getting the physiological signals that something exhilarating was going on. I had found a new thrill.

I see this exhilaration on my daughters' faces when they
visit the playground—the joy and the adventure. Siena climbs
bravely to the top of the jungle gym and then slides down, gig-
gling and grinning ear to ear. Sophie is in her version of heaven,
immediately running toward the monkey bars. When she first
started kindergarten, she was hardly able to jump and reach the
first bar without falling to the (thankfully cushioned) ground
below. But that girl is determined. Now, she proudly shows me
the pink calluses on her palms, evidence of her hard work to get
herself across those bars. Today she can skip two bars at a time
and dismount with a flip.

Yoga is my playground. I'm building up my calluses. Every
time I practice yoga I experience novelty; I am learning something new, inching my body toward new boundaries, and
taking risks. In yoga, I get those jumping-out-of-an-airplane
feelings, despite being firmly rooted to the ground.

I continued to show up for those Level Two classes and noticed that my body was rapidly changing; I felt stronger, more
flexible, and had noticed a sense of lightness and openness.
Then one day my instructor asked me if I had learned the "closing sequence" to the practice, which I hadn't yet. He talked me
through the various postures—including the wheel, shoulder
stand, plow, flying fish, and ending with the "king of all poses,"
the headstand.

Going upside down? The thought of it scared me. I had
tried headstands a couple of times earlier in my life, precancer,
always against a wall for support. But in my studio, I'd never
seen anyone use the wall. The goal was to build up strength

and balance in modified poses first, and eventually rise into that upside-down king of all poses without needing a prop or support.

Despite my fear, I let my teacher assist me into a headstand: my forearms pressed firmly in a V-shape around my head into my mat, my torso and legs shooting up above me. The instructor held my legs up straight. My head felt a rush of blood and my arms and shoulders were clenched tighter than they had ever been in my life. I felt like a tensed-up fist. The instructor moved his hands (just slightly) away from my legs for a moment and I felt a surge of a swooshing sensation through my body—according to my teacher, this is the feeling of finding one's balance upside down. I immediately brought my feet and legs down to the safety of my mat.

"How was that?" the instructor asked me.

I think that he expected me to say something like "Great!" or "Interesting!" Instead, I replied, "That was really terrifying," my eyes wide with anxiety. I knew that I was *not* going to go upside down again anytime soon.

The upside-down unsteadiness triggered petrifying memories of physical instability, when my balance was nonexistent during those walker-assisted cancer days. I remembered not being able to trust my body's ability to follow my brain's commands. Upside down, I felt a rush of trauma-triggered panic, and the catastrophic thoughts started to mount: *I could fall! If I fall sideways, I could snap my neck! What about those nonbone bones of mine? Would they shatter? If I get an injury, will I be confined to my bed again for who knows how long?* I felt completely out of control.

Posttraumatic stress symptoms have a way of staying quiet—

suggesting that perhaps all has been healed, that the trauma has determined its home is no longer to its liking, and has packed its bags and gone elsewhere. Forgetting all my clinical training, I had convinced myself that my trauma had been processed—as if my cancer history and memories had been neatly filed away in their respective bins in my brain and wouldn't need to be looked at again. But it's not that simple. In the face of significant triggers, which for me (and for many) are physical sensations, the trauma-induced panic comes roaring back. It surprises me when it shows up again, since I've had longer and longer intervals of feeling mostly recovered from my previous trauma-stricken state.

I walked home from that headstand yoga class, deep in thought along Amsterdam Avenue. I have always loved a challenge, and yoga had provided me with so many in a playful, inspiring way. But I felt like I had hit a wall. Should I, given my nonbone bones, steer clear from going upside down in yoga? Is it idiotic to even consider the pose? Could this be a physical limit that I should just respect and make peace with the notion of staying upright? Or is going upside down akin to my previous pursuit of touching my toes—something that seems unattainable but is actually possible? Maybe it's just my trauma-triggered, misguided fear that's holding me back from my potential to safely go upside down? I recognized my fixation on the headstand was my attempt to rebel against the cancer, to position my body into shapes that I had never aspired to even before the diagnosis.

By the time I got home, I had decided to work on the modified poses slowly and see how it felt to try easier versions of the headstand. But most importantly, I would hire my yoga instructor for a one-on-one lesson to get the emotional and physical support I needed to learn this new, terrifying posture.

In our first private session, I briefly went up into a crouched-ball version of a headstand. It felt much safer to have my knees tucked in, close to my body, as opposed to sticking up straight into the sky against gravity. I still clenched my whole body and felt afraid, but I was not out-of-control panicked. This was progress.

My instructor and I planned to meet for a few more sessions to work on the headstands together, but I kept having to cancel because I continued to get sick with some sort of wintery cold or respiratory infection. But on the days when I felt well enough, I would enter that knee-bent headstand position on my own, holding it for maybe five seconds, then ten seconds, and weeks later, fifteen. I imagined that with continued practice, my body would become more accustomed to being upside down, and would be less likely to erupt into a panic response.

I continued to give my brain and body the message that it's OK for me to be upside down in that little crouched-ball position. But I decided to wait to lift my legs until I had an expert by my side to assure me that it was safe for me to challenge both my mind and body to feel the unsteadiness, and find my balance in the unfamiliar.

PART V

INTEGRATION

37

INFORMED DENIAL

In my attempts to increase my sense of control over a mostly-out-of-my-control situation, I sought out all sorts of lifestyle changes that have been associated with reduced cancer mortality. It's not surprising that cancer patients experience a higher rate of anxiety, depression, and general symptoms of psychopathology as compared to their healthy peers.[1] Tragically, this shift in mood can be a literal killer. According to research, depressed cancer patients' chronically elevated stress states are associated with immunosuppression (interference with the body's antitumor cell activity), gene modulation (reduction in normal tumor suppressant gene functioning), and an increase in cancer invasiveness.[2, 3] These adverse effects of untreated depression are correlated with a quicker death.[4] To hopefully avoid becoming one of those statistics, I've added supportive interventions to my armory to bolster me physically and psychologically, including acupuncture, a plant-based diet, therapeutic massage, vitamins and supplements, my own psychotherapy, and yoga.

At times, people ask me if I've considered joining a support group. Support groups can be an excellent antidote to isolation, especially for "at risk" populations, such as cancer patients.[5] Groups can also serve as a preventative intervention for those who may be functioning well psychologically right now, but are vulnerable to significant emotional distress in the future. In fact, researchers have found that self-compassion, social support, and a sense of belonging increase resilience among breast cancer patients—and a group is an excellent modality in which to boost the above variables.[6]

As a psychologist, I've facilitated many a group. For those who have difficulty communicating their hurt, a group can offer opportunities to begin to experiment with self-expression in a safe, validating environment. Participants often learn that their experiences are not strange, and as a result, they feel less shame. It can be incredibly moving to be a member of a community and realize: I'm not the only one who's been having these thoughts and feelings—we are in this together and can help each other through it.

Luckily, I was not struggling from a depressive episode or an anxiety disorder after my breast cancer diagnosis. I was, however, experiencing a reduction in my quality of life, physical pain, and bouts of trauma-related symptoms, sadness, and worry. Perhaps group membership in a setting that promoted social and emotional connection with the underlying mutual understanding of living with this crazy disease could be of use to me. Maybe injecting my life with additional belongingness would protect me from the possibility of depressive and/or anxiety symptoms in the future.

Despite my knowing full well about the advantages of support groups, I was reluctant to actually attend one. They didn't appeal to me, though I wasn't sure why. Maybe because I provide therapy for a living? Maybe a (misguided and narcissistic) part of me believed that, given my profession, I already knew what would be learned in a group? I thought my time would be better spent at the yoga studio or chatting with a friend. But in my "I'll try anything" approach to fighting the cancer, on a sweltering day in July 2018 I dragged myself to my first meta-static breast cancer support group.

As I rode the subway downtown to the meeting, I couldn't help but think, What am I getting myself into? I exited the station in Chelsea, located the building, and made my way up to the metastatic breast cancer support group to find eight women seated at a large, rectangular table. As my eyes made their way around the table, I found myself thrust back into my fixation on hair. Each woman's hair (or lack thereof) seemed an indication of her stage of illness. There were bald women whom I labeled as actively in treatment receiving chemother-apy. A long-haired woman, who I'd learn was eight years out from her last chemo dose. There were wigs on other women's heads, but the lack of eyelashes and eyebrows revealed their af-fliction. Perhaps the saddest of all—there was one woman with long beautiful hair, who had just been diagnosed and had not yet started treatment. She was at the very beginning of this or-deal. She seemed so brave to me. I wouldn't have been able to show up at a group during that early phase of my illness. Back then, I took information in as was necessary; I wasn't looking for elaboration. But there she was, sitting in a room with the realities of her diagnosis—three months out, eight years out—all around her.

I smiled as I made eye contact with each of the group mem-bers and made my way to a chair. Sitting next to me was a young woman in her thirties. I recognized myself in her face, that telltale Herceptin light pink rash. She, I would learn that day, had been diagnosed with Stage IV cancer at a foreign hospital while on her honeymoon. It turns out that there are a lot of shitty ways to be diagnosed with cancer.

The group facilitator asked us to share how we'd been doing, and we went around the room, each taking our turn. There were stories of physical pain; fear, disappointment, and rage that treatment wasn't stalling tumor growth; realizations that one's marriage was not going to survive the cancer. With each person's sharing, I felt comforted to be in a room with women who totally "got" this whole cancer thing. But there was another part of me that wanted to run for the hills.

I was seated second to last in the storytelling line. When it was my turn, I summarized my cancer history in a six-sentence paragraph, covering the basics: I was pregnant when the cancer was initially detected; diagnosed with metastatic disease pretty much hours before giving birth to my baby; couldn't walk from the bone lesion pain; had a super-response to treatment; now am NED and continuing immunotherapy; and trying to figure out what the hell just happened. There was silence and deep respect as I spoke. The women were welcoming, empathic, and kind.

But I didn't feel like I fit in. I heard story after story of women trying new chemotherapy agents, and the cancer continuing to grow. Another was trying to get into an upcoming clinical trial for an alternative drug, in hopes that it could suppress the raging disease. How could I shed tears at that table, as an NED-er, while there were women who were dying all around me? There was one other NED patient in the room. She was a regular in the group and was able to share her vulnerability openly. Nobody seemed to be judging her or her distress. There was no evidence to suggest that the group members thought that I should leave their table.

Maybe they picked up on my discomfort, because some started to share with me, "I was NED, too, for [*seven weeks, four months, two years*] and now the cancer is back again, so we're all in the same boat." So maybe I did deserve a spot at that table, after all. But fuck. I didn't want to be in that boat!

As the thoughts swirled around in my head about NED, worthiness of being in the group, and what seemed like the inevitability that the cancer would come back at any second, I also noticed that I was having a difficult time taking my clinical hat off. I felt an internal tug of war between being a patient and a psychologist, and I couldn't figure out how to just be a group member. I noticed a woman in her early twenties. She was so quiet. I wanted to hear her voice, and to honor her spot in the room with the rest of us. Was that a clinical longing, or simply a human impulse to connect with another person? I felt like I was sitting on my hands, trying to keep myself from tinkering with the group through my own interventions or caretaking. All in all, I was *not* a present participant in that group session.

Toward the end of the meeting, the facilitator made mention of the women who were not in the group that day. They were not absent because of scheduling conflicts or treatment-related issues. They were not at the table because they had died earlier that year. She said the names of the two women that the group had lost, and there was a moment of silence. Some members started to tear up, while others wept. I sat there, taking it all in, thinking, Jesus, this is pretty dark.

The group meeting came to its end, and we all parted ways. I thought, One and done. No more support group sessions for me. It's just too intense.

Then I started to wonder. Why was I avoiding an experience that had the potential to promote my well-being? Psychology research tells us that anxiety-provoking situations generally become tolerable as our bodies and brains habituate. Did I just need more time, more exposures, to adjust to the new, challenging setting? To the reality that we all will die in time, for some of us it's just sooner than for others? I wasn't sure whether I should listen to every bone in my body that screamed, "Never go back!" But since I worried that I could be missing out on an important part of my healing and recovery, I decided to give the group another try.

The next session was crowded with more women and new faces, though I took the same seat as I had the time before and found some comfort in that one bit of familiar. There was a different group facilitator, and she had a more hands-off approach. There was no around-the-room check-in. Women spoke when they were inspired to do so. At times, I felt engaged and drawn in by the women and their vulnerability. But for the most part I experienced the group as chaotic and unpredictable. There were also complex interpersonal dynamics playing out in the group that day. One of the women spoke the majority of the time, repeating that she had it worse than everyone else in the room. The rest of the women appeared to be silenced by her message.

I wanted to bolt out of that room as fast as I possibly could. Between the intensity of the first group meeting and the out-of-control feeling of the second, I decided, I gave it an honest try. And after that, I didn't go back ever again.

But I remained on the email chain with all of the group members. At first it felt comforting to be a part of a cancer community, to support one another virtually. But soon after I stopped attending the in-person sessions, I noticed that when I received a new group email, marked in bolded black on my computer or cell phone screen, my heart would start to beat a little faster and my chest would tighten. I was bracing myself for the words I was about to read. Maybe it would be good news, like congratulating a member who had just run a marathon, against the impressive odds. Maybe it would be planning for the next potluck—who would bring what dish. But it was the other emails—the ones about treatments failing, tumors continuing to spread, the potential for needing amputation. My mind started to spin after reading those emails about the illness taking over, having no mercy for these beautiful people and the beautiful lives they so wanted to live. I realized it may be avoidance, but I couldn't be on that email thread anymore.

I contacted the group facilitator and explained that the emails were too emotionally overwhelming, that I was unable to participate in the group, and to please remove me from the list. She responded sensitively and asked me to reach out if I changed my mind down the line. I still get an email every now and then, someone responding to an earlier thread that I had originally been "CCed" on. I don't engage. I delete the email while it's still in bold, an unopened message that I will never read.

There is another potential explanation for why I had such a hard time with the metastatic breast cancer group. My profession requires that I listen to and help my patients process the most painful, scary, and vulnerable parts of their lives and selves, and I am with my clients 100 percent as they share their suffering with me. Therapists who work with traumatized clients need to be mindful of the risk of becoming "vicariously traumatized," which refers to when a therapist experiences trauma symptoms as a result of hearing, in vivid detail, the horror stories that can be people's realities.[7] I had never experienced vicarious traumatization to date in my practice, but perhaps that metastatic group setting was my first taste of it. My whole life, professional and personal, was trauma, and sitting in that room surrounded by so many traumatized women, I had reached my trauma limit.

There is no one-size-fits-all for self-care. In my psychology practice, I meet my patients where they are. Some are ready to unpack their trauma history after just a handful of sessions working together. Others need years to be able to do just that. I may need more time before I'm able to tolerate the discomfort that took over when I was in those support group sessions or reading the group emails. Or maybe I already have a sufficient dose of social support in my life right now, and my family and friends are all I need to bolster myself psychologically and physically. Perhaps I am even practicing self-care by limiting my dose of trauma and am protecting myself from vicarious traumatization.

My late godmother, who had lived with Stage IV breast cancer for many, many years, shared with me that her secret to coping with the disease was *informed denial*. I love this phrase. It perfectly sums up how I want to go about living my life. Yes, it's a fact that I could shift from NED status to a tumor-ridden patient at any time. But why think on that thought? There isn't much utility or comfort in that notion. Though I'm typically not pro-denial, in the case of my NED cancer, I think it works pretty nicely. I stay informed: I attend all of my doctors' appointments; my body is scanned; my blood evaluated. But the rest of the time, I try to focus on the present moment as opposed to the "what if," future-focused worry thoughts.

Maybe one day I'll go back to a cancer support group. Maybe it will be enormously beneficial for me at a different time in my life. But for now, I'll continue along in my informed denial, and remain a support group dropout.

38

WHAT'S NEXT

During the final stage of trauma recovery, the mind is now able to integrate traumatic memories because of its "innate tendency" to make sense of the senseless through cognitive flexibility and "complexity."[1] This complexity in cognition creates space for the more brutal facts of life: death is inevitable; there are inherent limits to our capacities; and at times, terrible things can happen to us. Although these facts were initially completely overwhelming, they are no longer a source of hopelessness or despair. Survivors have learned that life can deal us awful blows but—after necessary mourning and processing—we can return to living fully, and even with joy.

In what feels like being released from the shackles of intrusive thoughts, the terrifying incident is no longer played on loop at the forefront of your mind. Initially, our traumatic memories are like splintered sensory glimpses that erupt without warning.[2] At this phase of trauma recovery, however, these scattered recollections are gathered and then strung together to create meaning. This has likely occurred after the arduous and brave work of remembering one's trauma and sharing it with a trusted confidant. The act of truth-telling, to oneself and others, often results in reduced shame, fear, and feelings of loss, and provides the opportunity to advance forward and create new memories.[3]

When you are no longer alienated from yourself, others, and the world, there is now a profound sense of relief that life can be lived with delight and a newfound freedom. Like Sylvia Fraser, a survivor of childhood incest as described in Judith Herman's groundbreaking book on trauma, you may even feel a new vitality, as if you have suddenly "burst into an infinite world full of wonder."[4] No longer living in the past, you are actively engaged in the present and—for the first time in your new post-trauma life—feel hopeful for the future.

I have a complicated relationship with my body. Sometimes, it is my teammate—cooperating with me as I move through yoga poses or the impromptu dance parties with my children in our living room. But much of the time, I now experience my body as a container that is separate from my *self*. I'm still living here in it, but it's become clear that my body's time is finite, that it can only carry me for so long. I had been angry with my body for not keeping me protected, for breaking what I perceived to be a tacit agreement. But eventually I realized that my body never made me any promises.

Unconsciously, I took stock of the statistics and integrated them into my life assumptions. The average life span. The improbable tragedy of having a stillborn or being in a plane crash. Those numbers—however big or small—lent a false sense of safety. And when my body went in the direction of the outlier numbers, I felt betrayed.

But I don't feel betrayed today. It is a miracle, what my body has been able to achieve, even before its extraordinary response to cancer treatment. I am made up of more than thirty trillion cells. When I breathe one of the over twenty thousand breaths I inhale each day, the oxygen-rich air travels through my nose and mouth, down my esophagus, into my lungs, and then that oxygen is carried via my bloodstream to support the various organs of my body—my heart, which continues its steady beat, that tireless drummer. My body is held steady and in balance from tiny sensory neurons in my ear and the stretch receptors in my muscles and ligaments. Those sensory neurons and stretch receptors are so far away from each other, yet somehow they work together to keep me upright. When I want to move, my muscles contract in response to my brain's signaling some of its eighty-five billion nerve cells. How intricate, complex, and impressive our bodies are! I'm not angry with my body anymore; it's trying the best it can and has provided me with a pretty comfy home for many years.

Back in 2018, I carried the weight of my cancer diagnosis with me everywhere I went. There was never a moment when the word CANCER wasn't taking up essential real estate in my brain. I felt caged in by that word, by the meaning it carried, the notion of potential being stripped away.

Today, cancer is no longer in caps or in bold. When the word pops up, I usually don't feel the hopelessness, the sadness, or the loss that I needed to feel earlier in my recovery. Now I am able to walk with ease; there is pep in each step, the exciting sense of possibility. And I actually choose to hear that word, putting in my earbuds as I listen to my favorite song, "Near Death Experience Experience," by Andrew Bird:

And we'll dance like cancer survivors
Like your prognosis was that you should've died . . .

And we'll dance like cancer survivors
Like we're grateful simply to be alive

Although once sick, my living body is one to be celebrated. I sometimes get lost in my amazement for how much it has given me. But my girls, and their being brought to life in my body, is the most astonishing, mind-blowing gift of all.

Though one day, I'm not sure when, I will die. That is a fact. I do not fear death, but I do fear how my death will impact the people in my life if my time comes up well short of that average life span number. I desperately want to stay put, first, for the sake of my children, and second, because I happen to really enjoy living this life of mine.

It would be comforting if I imagined that when I die, I would ultimately be reunited with my loved ones. But I don't believe in an afterlife. It's perhaps not the most inspiring theory, but I expect that when I die, there will be an end, not another beginning.

How do I want this body to be handled when I die, once the "I" of "me" no longer resides within this flesh or is held up by these bones? When my organs have ceased their hard work, all in unison, of trying to maintain the equilibrium of such a complicated being with so many necessary parts? I envision that when I die, the intangible part of me that comprises my selfdom will float out of my body, tiny bubble-like wisps that will eventually dissipate up into the ether.

I can be set on fire. I am drawn to the idea of taking up less physical space to make more room for the living (plants count, too). But my experience with cremation has been limited to the movies, where there's always some sort of mishap. I hope that if I am cremated then my ashes could be scattered, without major hiccups, at my favorite nature preserve. There's an opening after being in the deep woods, and all of a sudden the hiker is standing at an inlet, marshland surrounding it, and in the distance, a vast harbor. Sometimes an egret can be found in the cove, slender and graceful, a dramatic white against the darker blue of the water. But I hear that scattering ashes into nature can harm delicate ecosystems, which is the last thing I would ever want to do with my remains. Scrap that idea.

Then there's the ground. Is there enough space for me in the earth? I would hate to take away any precious, untouched earth we have left and dig it up just for my body. Though there are "green" burials now—perhaps that can be my last wish. That there be a purchased patch of nature that is protected from turning into yet another strip mall or parking lot. I like the idea of becoming part of that dirt, deep down, closer to where the tree roots start to embrace into a world of entanglement, stretching farther than we can imagine when simply viewing what looks to be just one tree.

Please, do not embalm me with chemicals. Let my body carry on with its natural decay. Wrap me in a cotton shroud, like I am a present to the earth. Place me deep in the ground. Let my body feed the plants and animals, as they have fed me. Let me become a small part of those tree roots, nourishment to the leaves that grow from that root to trunk to branch, finally reaching with determination into the sky.

Make it a place my children and their children can visit and feel my presence around them, a preserved piece of land that awakens the senses of sight, smell, touch, and sound. Perhaps those visitors, if they do come, will feel the sturdiness of the earth and know that I am in the soil beneath their feet, and can be conjured up to remind them of their resilience.

I hope that the moments I've shared with people throughout my life have made some sort of positive difference, maybe if just to a handful of people. I like to imagine that those interactions have created meaningful interpersonal marks, like invisible tattoos, with traces that have the potential to be carried down to future generations. So perhaps I will live on in a way through my relationships. It's not heaven, but it's something.

39

THE OTHER BIG C

On the days that aren't too cold and rainy, I take myself for a walk outside along the country road, passing the trees still waiting to bud, the marshland, and the wide open, unobstructed sky. Despite the beauty all around me, there is an eerie quietness. I walk by the big gray house where the teenage boy plays basketball by himself, every day, alone with his ball, thump-thump-thumping. I wonder, When will he have a friend to play with him? Yesterday, I saw a fifty-something-year-old woman picking up trash on the side of the road. She was not a sanitation worker, just an eco-minded, kindhearted citizen. And today, I smiled in appreciation as I noticed that the grass along my daily walking route was litter-free.

Life has changed pretty dramatically. I am no longer in New York City. In March 2020, I packed up my family, and for the first time ever, was not sure when we would be coming back home. We are hunkering down on Shelter Island, waiting for our city, and our world, to recover from the coronavirus pandemic—the new big C.

I bet that the coronavirus and cancer would be best friends, if those little cells knew how to form companionship: they have much in common. They are both invisible. We can't see cancer or the virus with our naked eye, but we know that they exist. Their presence manifests as a constant hum in the background, engulfing us in fear and uncertainty.

When we first arrived at my parents' home on Shelter Island, I would look out all around me—surrounded by breathtaking nature, my children's delighted faces—but there was always something holding me back from fully enjoying the moment. It was my heart. It was beating faster, in what felt like a 50 percent increase from its normal rate, constantly keeping the same quickened rhythm, in the background of every scene from waking in the morning until lying down to sleep at night.

I couldn't remember ever having that kind of chronic, elevated anxiety plant itself in my chest and my heart. During the cancer diagnosis crisis period or the subsequent trauma-triggered panic attacks, my heart rate spiked but then normalized within minutes or hours. But on the island I was riding an elevated wave of anxiety that seemed as if it would never reach its crest and fall.

A jumble of thoughts whirled around my head, predominantly attempts to problem-solve my current situation. Since I had started cancer treatment, it became glaringly clear that I no longer had the capacity to care for my kids on my own, full-time. There is a required physical stamina to parenting that I just don't have. How would I ensure care for my children, and by extension, for myself?

Childcare is such a loaded issue for me. It's all tangled up with societal expectations, my own fantasies of what I anticipated I would be like as a mother, and the resultant shame of my believing that I don't measure up to my own yardstick of mothering success. I know, rationally, that I was dealt a tough hand, and that my cancer diagnosis and treatments have real consequences in terms of what I am and am not able to do in all facets of my life. But its invisibility—you can't *see* the fatigue— is what makes it that much harder. It's not like walking around with a broken arm and people know not to hand you bags of groceries. Sometimes, because of the side effects' invisibility, even I question whether I am just making too big a deal out of my physical limitations and *should* (there's that mean word again!) just toughen up and get it all done. But when I push myself too far, I end up in bed for days thereafter, trying to recover.

We had agreed that our babysitter would come out for the first Monday-through-Friday workweek and then reassess as we got more information about COVID-19 and New York City's response to it. With our girls cared for, I was able to go for a walk by myself, though it felt like I had this constant, highstrung companion in tow. I just couldn't get a break from that racing heart. The sun was starting to set as I made my way back to the house, pinks, blues, and oranges lighting up the sky. And I was on my way to a full-on panic attack.

I got upstairs, hidden away from the kids, and started to sob, my torso heaving with each attempt to bring in air. I couldn't figure out what to do. How could I protect all of us from getting sick, either from COVID-19 or me from sheer exhaustion and stress? I felt a mixture of shame and terror, knowing that I didn't have the physical strength to care full-time for my kids, and that my body would enter a state of utter collapse if I tried. And then I realized, there was a thought just above the surface of my conscious awareness that I was starting to get a view of, and it went something like this: *I tried so hard to stay alive, and now this virus is going to get me. And if I get the coronavirus, I will die.*

This was all starting to make sense. My anxiety was not just the body's natural response to being in the middle of a pandemic (anxiety in the face of the unknown is adaptive); it was also mixed in with my history of nearly dying from a disease and being vulnerable to and therefore understandably frightened of illnesses. Nothing like a pandemic to trigger a trauma reaction, drawing helplessness memories out front and center.

Trauma recovery is an ongoing process, one that never reaches the equivalent of a storybook's "The End." Environmental and body sensation triggers are muted, but they are never erased; so trauma-panic reactions, though less frequent or debilitating, may still arise.[1] My attempts at engaging in a headstand is an example of a trauma-triggering scenario that elicited emotional, cognitive, and physiological symptoms. These symptoms are normal and are not indicative of "backtracking." During this final stage of trauma recovery, survivors have a fuller understanding and appreciation for their trauma history, are less terrified by the body's feeling states, and are able to recognize, label, and anticipate these reactions accurately. The trauma is viewed through an empowered lens, and there is deep comfort in knowing, from ample experience, that these uncomfortable moments both make sense and are temporary.

I notice my trauma-panic symptoms surface when I mistakenly glance at metastatic breast cancer mortality rates without first preparing myself, with deep breaths, for the statistics—even though I already *know* the numbers, and I remind myself that I am not just a statistic, seeing them in print is consistently alarming. I also recently experienced trauma-induced panic while showering. Feeling warm and safe under the steady stream of water, I realized that soon I would have to leave the stall and brave the cold air of the bathroom. I had a flashback to the chemo-induced menopause symptoms, my evening routine of what felt like a million icicles piercing through my already freezing flesh. In clear contrast to the trauma reactions of the early recovery days, I was able to recognize my distress— momentary stilted breathing and increase in heart rate—as a result of my trauma *history*. And then refocus on the present moment.

But the coronavirus didn't feel like something I could shake off as easily. I thought to myself, OK, trauma, here you are. So now what? I evaluated the evidence to support and refute my notion that if I contracted coronavirus, I would die. Yes, I am in the "higher risk" category. But just because I'm higher risk does not mean that if I get coronavirus, there is a 100 percent chance that I will die. I would reduce my exposure the best I could, but I would also have to accept that there was a chance that I, like all people, could get COVID-19. And we would deal with that reality if it were to arise. There were no guarantees of a specific outcome. This was familiar uncertain territory, and we would be able to navigate it again, as we had ever since the cancer diagnosis two and a half years prior.

I also upped my self-care as best I could. My appetite had taken a nosedive, but when I could stomach it, I indulged in ice cream festivities with Derek and the girls. I had three sessions with my therapist over the span of ten days (a major increase in frequency after meeting with her for monthly boosters only). I practiced yoga when I could, some days for an hour, other days for five minutes. Derek had found our old CD collections stowed away in the back of a closet, and used my parents' stereo (circa 1990) to blast our favorite songs from our teens and twenties for family dance parties.

Most of all, I cuddled my girls. I remember when Siena had been sick with croup when she was eighteen months old, and her little stomach was rising and falling rapidly in retractions as she tried, with difficulty, to breathe. At the ER, she was given medicine and her breathing returned to normal. In order to be discharged, the hospital needed to get a heart rate reading below a certain mark, but every time the nurse applied the Band-Aid-like pulse sensor to Siena's big toe, she started wailing, and her heart rate shot up. When I scooped her up into my arms and held her against my chest, the sensor machine indicated a dramatic drop in Siena's pulse rate. Snuggled up next to me, she immediately calmed down. That sensor machine was the sweetest evidence of the effects of a parent's physical comfort on a baby's physiological arousal.

Like Siena, my heart rate had been above a reasonable cutoff mark. But when I held my girls, especially in the darkness of their rooms at the end of the days, I could feel the tension in my body release. I know that I was getting a surge of oxytocin— the "love" hormone that's released when you are intimate with someone you care for. That rush of warmth and connection gave my panicked body a much-needed break, and I relaxed so deeply, I nearly found myself falling asleep with my girls.

40

THE RED PLAID SHIRT

There are people who live through wars. They don't know where or when the next bomb will be detonated. Uncertainty and danger are entrenched in daily living. I do not know that kind of trauma, that kind of disaster. There was a war of sorts against COVID-19, but I was not at the front lines like the nurses and doctors and grocery store workers. I know how lucky I was to be in the safety of my parents' house in the country, to be able to settle into a quarantine routine.

When I first arrived on Shelter Island, the town's school had just canceled in-person classes. At the big hill along my walking route, teenage boys had taken over the empty road, practicing their skateboarding tricks when they used to be in algebra. But a few days later, they were gone. When I walked up or down that hill, I thought of those boys; presumably they were shut up in their respective houses, unable to hang out and explore normal teenage mischief together. I felt sad for them, to be missing out on relationships when friendships mean everything, shaping one's sense of self (I am/am not like this person) and providing necessary separation from parents. Those defined pockets of independence—skateboarding down the hill—are so central to healthy adolescent development.

When the boys disappeared, I realized that I should establish roots in our temporary home, too. The drawers and closets were full of my parents' clothes, and mine were lying in stacks on the floor. Each time I came into the bedroom, I saw the piles and was reminded that I was in a state of flux, like living out of a suitcase. It was time to make some room, to get my clothes off the floor, and give myself permission to stay in my new borrowed home for a while.

I opened my father's closet and there, resting perfectly on its hanger, was the red plaid shirt. It was my mom's oversize shirt, the one she had given me when I was first diagnosed with cancer, my body huge with Siena growing inside me. With the buttons undone, I got an extra layer of warmth that almost fit my large belly. After I gave birth to Siena, that shirt stayed with me still and remained my daily uniform as I started cancer treatment. It became a protective barrier, a cozy companion, a representation of my mother's love wrapped all around me. I wore that shirt when I was on the walker—when I was at my sickest and dying—and as I started to gain back my strength and the potential to live again.

One year out from my diagnosis, when I was no longer in the throes of illness, I purged my closet of maternity clothes and it was with mixed emotions that I gave the red plaid shirt back to my mother.

Yet there was the shirt again, hanging at the ready to be worn during the next crisis: this time, the coronavirus pandemic. I studied the garment—the predominantly red plaid crisscrossed with columns of green, blue, white, and yellow. The fabric was slightly faded, though when I considered that it had been worn for three decades, I was impressed by its brightness and heft. I put it on. It had the same cozy feeling, that same warmth it had provided during my cancer crisis. The shirt was way too big for me—I was swimming in it—but it felt just right.

The shirt has been a part of my life since I was about seven years old. It had originally been my brother's, then my mother's, and then for some reason it ended up in my father's closet. Mostly I remember the red plaid shirt on my mother, her looking so comfortable seated in the living room's armchair, either reading the *New York Times* or filling out the crossword puzzle, her sweet face dimly lit by the yellow glow of the table lamp beside her.

During the coronavirus days, I wore the shirt almost every day all over again. Siena played with the brown, bone-like buttons, all still sturdily in place. With the sleeves rolled up, I could see my black elastic hair band, back to its home around my left wrist. I hadn't cut my hair and I resembled the comedian Carrot Top (in shape and volume, not color), when I didn't gather it back into a half pony. I felt thankful for the shirt and for that hair band, and for the unruly mop of hair upon my head.

During my last prepandemic appointment with Dr. Dang in the winter of 2020, we had decided to push out my infusion to eight weeks, since I had been struggling with back-to-back infections, my white blood cell count consistently in the low range. We hoped that by April the cold and flu season would have passed and I would be able to ward off illnesses a bit better after a longer break from treatment. Due to the increased interval between infusions, my oncologist moved up my next PET/CT scan to check me for tumor growth.

So much for the thought that April 2020 would bring a reduction in contagious illnesses! In order to reduce the number of patients going into the hospital (and potentially bringing COVID-19 with them), scans and other nonessential appointments were canceled at the cancer center, so no PET/CT scan for me. I was rescheduled to receive my next infusion at my hospital's satellite location, closer to my parents' home on Shelter Island.

On treatment day, I felt my muscles tense up as I climbed into the front seat of the car. I was scared. Derek was driving me to a treatment center, and I had been sequestered at my parents' house for a month. At that point, the quarantine had had the positive consequence of my feeling healthier than I had the entire winter. The lack of exposure to germs brought home by me, my husband, or, most likely, my kids meant that I had been healthy for the whole month, a major break from my previous back-to-back respiratory infections. Even my girls were peculiarly healthy, making it a full twenty-eight days without those parallel-line runny nose drips. But with treatment, I knew that my body would undergo another inflammatory assault, and that I would be exposed to *other people* (have they been downgraded to potential virus carriers only?) outside of my immediate family for the first time. Would my seeking cancer immunotherapy result in my contracting the virus?

After arriving at the center, I passed the coronavirus screening test and was allowed up the elevator to the waiting room. As each patient was called in for treatment, I switched seats to expand my personal bubble (sometimes by only a foot or two, but it seemed a necessary addition). All of the patients were wearing masks, save for one elderly woman who kept her mask bunched up around her neck as opposed to her face. She coughed from time to time, and in my mind, each one sounded as if she were coughing into a megaphone. I tried to remind myself that I would be out of that waiting room soon. I told myself that it made sense that I felt anxious—I knew that I was increasing my risk of coming down with some bug, and possibly the coronavirus, just by sitting in that enclosed space. But I needed to stay put in order to receive the immunotherapy that keeps my cancer dormant. I would need to ride out this wave of normal, to-be-expected anxiety.

After an hour of my game of musical chairs around the waiting room, I was called back for treatment. All proceeded smoothly. My nurse was efficient and had no problem accessing my port. But over the course of my infusion, I was alerted that I had been in proximity to a person with COVID-19.

When I spoke with Dr. Dang the next day, she told me that if I had contracted the virus, the symptoms would, in all likelihood, arise within five days. Though unfortunately, she said, many of the side effects from Herceptin, my immunotherapy, overlap with COVID-19, so it would be difficult to determine whether my maladies were related to the medication or virus. Nevertheless, she told me to monitor my symptoms and to take my temperature daily.

As is usual after an infusion, for the next few days I was significantly fatigued. It was difficult to get out of bed. I could barely eat. My neck and shoulder muscles ached. I had a dry cough. My head felt as if there were a vise on the inside, positioned near my temples and ears, its gears in reverse, forcefully pushing out against my skull. I wondered—Is this Herceptin, or is this COVID-19?

Six days out from the infusion, I continued to be fatigued, though my appetite was starting to come back. The dry cough was infrequent, and I had no fever. The muscle soreness had largely subsided, though the head and ear pain remained. But with each passing day, I felt better. I was in the clear.

When my cancer was first diagnosed, I felt as if I were drowning in uncertainty. Now, in the time of coronavirus, the whole world is grappling with this unsettling reality of not-knowing.

The smallest things can make the most challenging of times just a little less overwhelming. For me, it was wearing my mom's red plaid shirt, wrapping it around me, to comfort me as I recovered from my infusions and as I wondered whether I had contracted COVID-19. With the red plaid shirt on, I felt a little safer. I felt a little calmer. I wasn't able to hug my mom, dad, or brother. But when I wore that shirt, I felt their embrace.

41

FAIRIES AND PORTS

One of my favorite moments of my day is around 7:00 P.M., when I lie down with my three- and seven-year-old daughters, often sandwiched between them, to read, sing, and snuggle before bed. It's an hour of relief and calm—we all made it there to Sophie's bed in one piece, to the end of the day. In all likelihood, it was a day full of fun and adventure, punctuated by minicrises like arguments about whose stuffy belonged to whom, the impassioned declarations of disinterest in the available meal and snack options, and possible tears to gently wipe off of little girl cheeks. But in the quiet of the bedroom, all of that falls away and we are aligned with the same goal of just being loving with one another.

Sometimes I read to the girls separately—Siena first and then into her crib she goes, and Sophie up next. Recently, I was lying next to Sophie in her bed, and reached over to her nightstand to pick up the new chapter book we were slated to begin: *Peter Pan*. I started reading, and immediately she asked me, "Mommy, are fairies real? Is the tooth fairy real?"

Sophie had lost many teeth over the previous months—she has that adorable gaping space where her two front top teeth are missing, and spaces beside her first two grown-up teeth in her lower row. The tooth fairy has been a frequent visitor to our home, working even during quarantine conditions. After waking one morning, finding crumpled dollar bills under her pillow, Sophie shared with me that she thinks there is one tooth fairy for about four different families so that the fairy doesn't get too worn-out. On the thrilling days when Sophie loses a tooth, she sits down and writes a letter to the tooth fairy. I save them all in a file, hidden away in hopes that Sophie will not find them until she is much older. One of them read:

my love tooth fary! I lost 3 tooths! and you'r gust amazing! gust the way you ara!

I'm holding on to the notion of Sophie as a little girl. She makes mistakes in pronunciation of certain words, like "aminal" for *animal* or "mines" for *mine*. I feel the internal tug to teach her the correct enunciation, but the part of me that wants to keep her little in my mind wins.

How was I supposed to respond to Sophie's question about the tooth fairy? It's not that she's been around other kids during the months of quarantine, who could have announced during recess that fairies and unicorns and Santa are all made up. This curiosity and inquiry are coming from Sophie.

So in an approach that at an older age she may find infuriating, I answered her question with a question.

"What do you think?" I asked.

Sophie replied, "I think you bring me the money at night."

I looked at her and smiled slightly, but her eyes did not meet mine. Sophie, her forehead slightly scrunched and eyes wide, was looking off into the space of her bedroom, clearly deep in thought. But I could see that she didn't have any more questions, and wasn't looking for me to either confirm or deny her hypothesis. So we went back to reading about the mischievous fairy Tinker Bell and Peter Pan's quest to remain a kid forever.

On the second night of reading *Peter Pan*, Sophie was snuggling up to me, she in an old T-shirt of mine, the fabric soft from decades of being washed, and me in my thin-strapped tank top and leggings. She placed her little fingers in that delicate recessed space at the base of my neck where my two collarbones meet. She noted the stickiness of my skin compared to hers (lotion, I explained), and continued to my right upper arm. And then in a very matter-of-fact way, she pointed at my right upper chest wall and said, "What's that, Mama?"

She was pointing to the lump on my upper chest—my port—the venous catheter that was implanted under my skin and attached to a vein to allow for the efficient and safe administration of chemotherapy and immunotherapy medications to treat my cancer. Lying so close to her, our heads touching, I felt a heaviness in what I imagined was my heart, but I was able to answer her questions.

"That's my port, honey."

"What's a port, Mommy?"

"A port is something that makes it easy for me to get my medications."

"How did you get the port?"

"I had surgery."

"What is surgery?"

"Surgery is when a doctor changes something about your body—Uncle Ben is a surgeon. The surgeon made a cut in my skin and then put the port there so I can get medicine easily."

"Did the surgery hurt?"

"No, they gave me medicine so that I didn't feel the surgery at all."

"What is it made of?"

"Huh, that's a good question. I'm not exactly sure. I imagine plastic and metal?"

"Metal!?!" Sophie laughed. "Was I alive when you got the port?"

"Yes, you were four years old."

"Was Siena alive?"

"Yes."

"Who took care of me and Siena when you had the surgery?"

"We had a baby nurse and your babysitter with you two—but Daddy and I came home from the surgery the same day so we weren't gone for long."

"Does it hurt when you get the medication in there?"

"Only the first second, but I don't feel it afterward."

"Does the medication make you tired?"

"Yes. You know how sometimes Daddy and I leave for the day for me to get my medication? That's when I get the medicine in my port. It makes me tired, so that's why I'm in bed a lot for the first few days after I come back from getting the medicine."

"Do all grown-ups have ports, Mama?" she asked.

"No, they don't."

"Am I going to have a port when I grow up, Mama?"

At this, my reasoned adult replies came to an abrupt halt. Tears streamed down my face as I replied, "No, sweetie."

Appearing to not notice the shift in my emotional state, Sophie pointed to the book, indicating that question time was over. And then back to *Peter Pan* we went, my eyes wet and my chest tightened with sadness and fear.

I didn't want to tell Sophie about the cancer. Yes, we had already had a conversation about it years ago, when she was four, but since I had become NED, it rarely came up. At times, I would ask Sophie if she remembered when I was sick, or on the walker, and she always said no. She remembered me having buzzed hair, and made it clear that it wasn't her preferred style for me.

Sophie is going to continue to question the stories that are presented to her—she's at that age now—the world of fantasy, make-believe, unicorns, and fairies is starting to be scrutinized. One day, she's going to ask me about why I get medication in my port and I will need to respond to her query without a question. I will need to tell her the truth. Luckily, I can tell her that I am NED, that I fought the cancer and won.

But I am so scared that this conversation will plant the seed that Sophie will lose me, and then she will carry that burdensome fear with her for the rest of my life. I remember having my own worries about my mother's death when I was a little girl, and my mom was healthy; I had no reason to worry about her untimely demise. During school theater classes I could immediately summon tears just by thinking about my mother dying one day. But Sophie would have a legitimate reason to be afraid. I almost died. And I am still fighting cancer.

I cried next to Sophie that night, but they were not simply sad tears. I was crying with gratitude to have the opportunity to have the port conversation with her to begin with. It wasn't a given that I would be alive this long to talk to my seven-year-old daughter about my port. It was with this mixture of emotions that I felt overcome by the gravity of our talk, its meaning, and thinking about the future—and the conversations that will come.

Like Sophie, before my diagnosis I lived in a sort of fairyland. I felt safe. I had the false assumption that I would never experience a life-altering and life-threatening trauma. But as if I were out at sea back in those days, in my innocence, my naivete, now I have been brought to shore. But it's still beautiful over here, even with the realities of life that are stripped of that fantasy. I continue to see magic all around me now—in these moments, I continue to be.

My trauma is still a part of me—its external representation is protruding from my chest wall, it's revealed when my emotions bubble over as I anxiously anticipate an upcoming PET/CT scan just weeks away. But I can live with this implanted device under my skin and with this trauma indelibly imprinted in my mind. I can honor my body's reactions, my tears, my joy and gratitude for being alive, my fear of not being around for my kids. I have a chronic illness, one I will be fighting for the rest of my life. I'm up for the fight.

42

LITTLE EARTHQUAKES

Most mornings, after I've digested my ritual breakfast of oatmeal with chia and berries, I perch my computer on top of my parents' floral love seat, lay out my yoga mat, and sign onto the Zoom yoga class with my teachers Jamie and Scott. In these "open" yoga sessions, I get to see my community as we practice postures at our own pace, confined to computer-generated squares like a Cirque du Soleil version of *The Brady Bunch* television show's opening credits.

I continued working on the upside-down modified headstand pose, my knees tucked in and the full weight of my body descending onto my forearms, during the coronavirus-friendly, virtual Ashtanga yoga classes. After months of hanging out in the crouched headstand, I was no longer tensing my muscles with all my might. There was an ease to the position that felt both unexpected and exciting. My yoga teachers told me that I was ready to lift my legs away from my torso to enter the "full expression" of the pose. But since they weren't physically by my side to hold me, they recommended that I set myself up next to a wall for support.

At this stage of trauma recovery, the accruing of trauma-contradictory experiences—perhaps by successfully asserting yourself in challenging interpersonal relationships or taking a kickboxing class—shifts your relationship with your body and self from helpless victim to empowered survivor. Body sensations and emotions are fully felt without dread or panic; a state of numb paralysis or hyperarousal is replaced with a state of color and vibrancy.

Here was another opportunity to support my newfound designation of my body as strong and able, which by extension would bolster my sense of self as strong and able, too. But attempting the headstand felt different from my initial postcancer diagnosis movement goal of touching my toes or twisting my spine. I wondered, Was this a completely stupid idea to try to go upside down without an instructor present?

I moved my laptop so that the camera angle displayed my whole body—as if my teachers' simply viewing me in full screen could prevent me from falling and breaking my back—and assumed that modified headstand with my thighs against my chest. Then I lifted my legs up into the air. In less than three seconds: I teetered forward and my heels made contact with the wall; I tried to move my feet; my weight shifted like a seesaw from my left to my right forearm; and then my legs landed behind me, ungracefully, with a loud thump onto the mat.

When I sat upright to face my teachers on the computer screen, I noticed that my brain felt heavy—a result of the inversion sending a rush of blood to my temples and forehead. My heart was beating from the physical exertion, but I was not in a panic; my nervous system was not triggered into a state of alarm. I said to my teachers, "I feel really wobbly, like I'm swaying from side to side. How can I keep my legs straight?" My teacher Jamie was the first to respond. "The swaying is part of the posture. Allow yourself to move slightly, shifting the balance around your base. Try not to grip—that's when you'll fall." My instructors then applauded my effort as an important first step toward finding comfort in this new, and historically very challenging (for me), pose.

Huh. So I was supposed to sway? I was baffled that allowing movement would actually maintain stability. I had the misguided notion that in order to balance, you need to stay absolutely still, like a statue. I thought that I was supposed to be impervious to wind, my children running around me in circles, and any other mental distraction or bodily sensation—that nothing should cause the solidity of my upside-down stance to waver.

Then I thought of those buildings in Japan and California that are built to withstand earthquakes by shifting with the movement of the earth's tectonic plates below them. Buildings with solid foundations embedded in the ground are more likely to topple over or crumble during an earthquake. To solve this problem, engineers invented "base-isolation structures," rubber-like foundations that absorb the shocks of the earth's movements, reduce structural shaking, and prevent collapse.[1] Like these new seismically safe buildings, I could also benefit from allowing my body's foundation to sway and responding to it gently, following it, and then ever-so-slightly moving in the opposite direction.

With my bizarre determination, every day, if I felt well enough, I attempted the full expression of the headstand. I noticed my body's subtle shaking—like little earthquakes—but I didn't clench up or try to fight the sway. I remembered when

I first attempted to go into the headstand during an in-person yoga class six months prior, when these quakes had completely overwhelmed my traumatized body and mind. The shakiness had triggered automatic, fear-laden cognitions that I would topple over and crumble. But now, I can notice the unsteadiness and move with it, not against it. I still feel hints of fear, though since it's been years since my cancer diagnosis, I have accumulated trust in my body and its ability, overall, to follow my brain's suggestions. Upside down, I respond to my body's cues, edging just a tiny bit more to the left, right, or center. It is like a dance with gravity.

After much practice, I'm now able to balance in a headstand for twenty-five seconds. I have moved away from the reassurance of the wall and enter headstands in the middle of rooms or outside in the grass. Following a recent blizzard, I planted my winter jacket-covered forearms and hat-protected head into the cold snow and assumed the posture, because, I wondered, What would it feel like to do a headstand in the snow? It felt like play. My hat-covered head and parka-covered forearms created an imprint into the white ground, and my upside-down body was gently held in place by the snow surrounding my foundation. I heard the subtle crunching sounds of the snow as my weight shifted. Then Siena, inspired to practice her own snow-day yoga, sidled up next to me and entered her favorite pose, the downward dog.

I experience a strange intoxication when I go upside down; my body craves it—the risk, the novelty—almost like a drug. But most of all, each time I go up into a headstand I feel enormously proud of my body. My self-imposed, gradual exposures to instability have transformed the sensation from terror and dread to one of fun and adventure. My body has come so far, from its cancer-induced reliance on a walker to hold me steady or being confined to bed, to today: I can walk; I can kneel down to the floor to play with my girls; I can skip along forest trails with my family. I have restored confidence in my body and in myself.

43

GOING HOME TOGETHER

In the early fall of 2020, our pandemic family ventured off Shelter Island to the nearby village of Greenport for an outdoor, socially distanced, coronavirus-compliant dinner. We were all giddy about our Japanese restaurant meal—our first since prequarantine days. Siena slowed us down by mindfully slurping each udon noodle in her soup, one by one, while the sun set and darkness settled in all around us. Long after Derek, Sophie, and I had finished our dumplings and maki rolls, Siena was still at work, intent on eating every last bite while the rest of us sat there, half-impatient, half-impressed.

Bellies full, we made our way back to the docks for our return to the island. Siena, not used to being outside in the dark, declared in her little three-year-old voice, "There are no lights!" and then asked, "Where are the lights?" with bewilderment and a hint of anxiety. I explained that we were outside at nighttime, that the sun had set, and that the moon was up in the sky—even though we couldn't see it through the overcast. Back in New York City, prequarantine, we were often out and about as a family in the evenings. But I realized that we hadn't been outside with Siena after dark for the past eight months, and she had apparently forgotten that at nighttime, there is darkness. I was surprised that in such a short time, Siena had cozied up to the idea that life is one big, long, sunshine-filled day.

While we waited for the ferry to arrive, a fog descended all around us, and we marveled at the way it played with the lights on buildings, spreading out the yellows, purples, and greens like a plump brush full of watercolor paint. Spotting the ferry in the water, we saw it approach us like an apparition hovering and mostly obscured by the clouds. It docked, let off its line of cars, and then we were directed by the captain to step aboard.

Off we went, floating on the water. All was black and blurred. There was wetness in the air, although it wasn't raining, and it looked and felt like there was a slick layer of water on everything around us. It was unclear how much the wetness was the result of the fog or the water from the bay. The sky and water had become one saturating entity, and we were moving through it.

The clouds were so dense that we could barely see ten feet ahead of us, and certainly not beyond the perimeter of the ferry. I wondered, How do the boats not crash into each other in this kind of weather? And then I got my answer. The ferry let out its foghorn—unexpected, loud, and steady. Like a tuba or other brass instrument, the horn's sound was deep and musical. Held for what seemed like at least five elongated seconds, the sound, urgent in its initial impact, slowly gave way and was carried across the water in what I imagined was a softer hum of warning.

Each time the horn blew, Siena, whom I was holding in my arms, jumped and looked all around her, stunned, wide-eyed, and trying to make sense of this extraordinary sensory experience. As I held Siena through the fog and her fear, her little head held erect instead of landing, at rest, upon my left shoulder, I caught sight of Sophie peering out into the darkness with her dad at the edge of the boat. For Sophie, this was a thrill, and she exuded both awe and excitement.

We approached an orange smear of light, and the closer we came to it the shape became smaller and slightly more in focus—turning out to be lights on the ferry slip we were expected to pull in to. The ferry captain managed to glide the large boat between the pilings, the parallel lines of branchless trees on either side of us.

We had gotten through the fog; we had made it to the other side. We stepped off the boat, from water onto dry land. And, like some miracle, we all went home together to our borrowed house on the island.

EPILOGUE

Before I started my writing experiment, I was lost in the world of my personal trauma. My perceived control over my disobedient body had vanished. I grappled with the real likelihood of dying and leaving my family, my girls—a newborn baby and a four-year-old—without their mom. I wanted to shield my seventysomething-year-old parents from the anachronistic misery of burying their own (adult) child. I felt identity-less, worried that I would forever remain an empty vessel, and never again experience joy, adventure, and the sweet eager anticipation that comes with living a full life.

My initial fear-encumbered thoughts, including that my trauma would result in a life sentence of psychological anguish, turned out to be completely inaccurate. What I didn't know, back in those days of what felt like a stuck point in my recovery, is that I had yet to meet the new me. All along, she was budding and stretching and doing the arduous work of beginning to make sense of the insensible.

The trauma didn't end when I received my NED status. It kept unfolding, in new iterations, as my body started to heal, then backtracked, then healed and backtracked again. I learned that this is the reality of living with a chronic illness.

Engaging in empowered body actions and writing made me whole again. Though my writing was initially intended to be an investigation into my past, it eventually became an exercise in the art of expressing that which was unfurling in the present—the pain and emotions that are a part of everyday living. My trauma narrative evolved into more than an exposure exercise to uncover memories from my traumatic past. Writing became medicine to help me cope with the uncertainty of the here and now. And perhaps the biggest surprise of all is that through the writing of my trauma narrative emerged my love letter to life.

By December 2020, I was putting the final touches on this manuscript with the goal to send it to agents at the beginning of the new year. But my project got sidetracked. My headaches were increasing in intensity and made it nearly impossible to think, let alone write. That vise-like sensation of gears pushing out into my skull was no longer confined to the days just after an immunotherapy infusion. The pain was constant and stubbornly unresponsive to medication.

On a Saturday in January 2021, I knew that my headaches had reached the "it's time to get this checked out" threshold. I felt a new pressure behind my right eye and noticed that my peripheral vision was off after repeatedly sideswiping cabinets and other furniture as I made my way around the house. After consulting with my cancer center's on-call doctor, Derek and I decided to drive into Manhattan the next day to get an MRI of my brain.

The evening prior to our trip, I started getting ready for sleep and was about to pull down the shade to the bedroom window, but for some reason I felt an urge to see the stars. So I craned my neck, tilted my head to the right, looking upward, and positioned my face against the windowpane. It was pitch-black save for the white stars that blanketed the sky, surprisingly bright and clear.

I stared at the stars and thought to myself, *After my doctor visit tomorrow, I don't think that the sky will ever look the same.* I thought the stars would be tainted somehow, that the sky would lose its magic, and life would be less beautiful. I wanted to pluck a star from the sky and put it in my pocket to somehow protect me from whatever the next twenty-four hours would reveal. As I continued to stare at the night sky I thought, *I'm so small. I'm less than a speck. And I think this speck's time may be up.*

The next day, while alone in the Urgent Care center due to COVID protocol, I was diagnosed with cancer in my lower brain. When my brain was first scanned back in October 2017, the cancer had already spread there but was "dormant" or "dust," and therefore not detectible. The treatments I've received over the years aren't able to pass the brain's blood-brain barrier, and so the cancer in my brain, once it woke from its dormancy, was able to grow and grow. Even my cancer blood markers, which have been in the low/normal range for years, haven't been able to access the cancer levels in the brain, which my doctors have aptly referred to as a "vault."

So back into survival mode I go. With this new diagnosis has come a whole new host of challenges: the manic episode I was launched into after taking high doses of steroids to reduce brain inflammation; deciding whether to discontinue my psychotherapy practice; navigating how to tell my seven-year-old and three-year-old daughters that mama has cancer in her brain.

But I have found deep comfort, this time around, knowing that I am on the familiar path of trauma recovery. This isn't my first rodeo, after all. My body and mind *need* to progress through the stages you've just read about in this book. I know that, while still real and still distressing, the fight-flight-freeze and betrayal will ultimately pass.

But I promised you, my beloved reader, a story of recovery. Can I still give that to you as I write these sentences with tumors in my brain? I always knew that the cancer could, and in all likelihood would, rear its head again. And in fact, I was never cancer-free. It's true that I may never recover physically from the cancer. But I *am* recovering from the cancer-induced psychological trauma.

The statistics, once again, are grim. At my inpatient hospital stay after the new diagnosis, one oncologist informed me that I had "two to three years" left to live. A social worker suggested that I start "legacy planning" and put together a "trinket box" for my daughters.

Perhaps I'm in denial. But I've landed on the notion that I was a statistical outlier in the past, and there's no reason to think that I won't be an outlier once again. Stephen Jay Gould, the famous evolutionary biologist and paleontologist, found himself in similar circumstances to mine many years ago when he was diagnosed with a rare and severe form of abdominal cancer. Upon researching his condition, he learned that the median (average) survival rate was eight months. But in his essay "The Median Isn't the Message," Gould interpreted this number with a scrutinizing eye, writing, "We still carry the historical baggage of a Platonic heritage that seeks sharp essences and definite boundaries."[1] He challenged the notion that means and medians, both measures of central tendency, can be viewed as "hard 'realities.'" Statistics, like everything else, are impacted by variability, by randomness. Gould ended up living twenty years beyond that eight-month average, and even died of another cause. We are creatures who crave certainty. But life, it turns out, is a study in uncertainty.

After receiving my new diagnosis, I made sense of another strange physical experience. In the month leading up to the brain MRI, I had been losing my balance in familiar, and previously steady, yoga poses. First, I teetered out of the more challenging postures, like the headstand, but then I started falling sideways out of simple lunges. It seemed odd, but I didn't make much of it at the time. I had finally come to a place of peace with those "little earthquakes" and was curious about, but not traumatically triggered by, my body's unsteadiness.

It turns out that those little earthquakes were not just the normal instability one would expect when attempting a challenging yoga pose. Those little earthquakes were actually triggered by the cancer tumors in my cerebellum, the brain region responsible for balance. As humans we sometimes worry about highly unlikely, worst-case scenarios. But I couldn't have manufactured this thought, that my shaking and teetering *were* in fact a herald of serious, life-threatening danger.

But the coping, whether it's a 2.0 or a 7.0 on the trauma Richter scale, remains the same. I am now, after recycling through the survival, betrayal, and dissociation phases of recovery, able to move with this shake-up, to accept that brain cancer is indeed my reality, and do, once again, everything I can to fight the disease. At this time of writing, I am happy to report my brain lesions have all reduced in size since the initial MRI scan in January. I am, as ever, hopeful.

In March 2021, high as a kite on steroids and obsessively cleaning my parents' home in Shelter Island, I found it difficult to make it outside for my daytime walks. The setting sun was the only alarm that could tear me away from my various "projects" and make me realize—your time's almost up, Sarah. Get outside. So I laced up my sneakers, Velcroed on the reflective wrist and ankle bands, and made my way to the country road. My walking in the dark became a recurring joke in the family, as every day I would wake up and state with authority, "Today I am going to make it outside while it's still light out!" But that day never came to pass while I was medicated on the steroids. In my persistent race against the sun, it inevitably grew dark. It was just me alone in the nighttime, walking with my flashlight in hand, and listening to the hooting owls along my route.

Sometimes I was so engrossed in tidying up that I got an extra-late start, the sun already slipping under the horizon. When the skies were clear I ended up walking beneath the stars. And I was right. About them never looking the same again. On one of those nights I stood in our gravel driveway for ten minutes, staring upward, and cried. Because the stars are more beautiful now than ever before.

Our lives are a collection of moments, some of them excruciating. But sidestepping the pain, the mourning, and the terror is an impossibility. We need to move through and with the despair, and give ourselves permission to feel, think, and sense *everything*, even in those moments of horror. Avoiding our internal experiences only leads to additional torment. We must try, with all of our might, to practice self-compassion as we navigate what will likely be the most grueling time of our lives, and hold close the knowledge that recovery lies just beyond the suffering.

If you have experienced a trauma, perhaps now you will pursue your own version of truth-telling—either in written or oral form—and actively engage in facing the past in an effort to engender healing. Our stories must be told. And we must find an active listener who will tenderly support the expression of our pain. Perhaps your listener is a friend, a partner, a family member, or a therapist. Rebecca Solnit writes, "To hear is to let the sound wander all the way through the labyrinth of your ear; to listen is to travel the other way to meet it."[2] Find and hold close those who will travel to meet you as you tell your story. Eventually, your narration will lead you into the present. There, you will be greeted by the gift of hope.

ACKNOWLEDGMENTS

My gratitude for the support in writing this book cannot possibly be summed up in a couple of pages; but nonetheless, I will try.

To Julia Kardon, agent extraordinaire. Thank you for believing in this project, selling it with all your might, and being devoted to my whole well-being from acquisition to print. Mary Gaule, my exceptional editor, thank you for your empathy and sagacity, which are equal in measure. To the fantastic team at HarperCollins, including Lydia Weaver, Shelly Perron, Becca Putnam, Kelly Doyle, Tina Andreadis, and the ever-supportive Sara Nelson. I will never forget our chance encounter at the Greenport bus-stop picnic tables, and for your generosity in reading the early pages of my book. Thank you to Jo O'Neill for the evocative and beautiful book cover and Leah Carlson-Stanisic for the delightful interior design. Harper has felt like a home from day one; thank you to everyone for welcoming me into what felt like a huge family hug.

To my friend and writing mentor Lisa Weinert, who convinced me that my book was meant to be read by others, gave me confidence in my "voice," and supported *Little Earthquakes'* first drafts. To my writer's group members who listened and responded to my stories with their entire selves. Thank you, Jennifer Kurdyla, for the editing and then virtually holding my hand over Zoom as I submitted the manuscript to agents. A big thank-you to all my early readers and their invaluable feedback and cheerleading—Barry Lubetkin, Val Monroe, Seth Fishman, Hala Alyan, Sam Klugman, Rachel Marlowe, Danielle O'Steen, and Jon Levy-Warren, among others.

Thank you to all of my doctors, nurses, and healthcare supporters at Memorial Sloan Kettering, especially Dr. Chau Dang. I am forever grateful to have you as my expert physician and be able to bask in the stunningly compassionate light you bestow upon me and, I imagine, so many others. You are a true gift to this world.

Thank you to my previous patients—I miss the incredible transformations I bore witness to in our work together. I hope that my writing serves as a reminder of my care and unrelenting trust in our ability to heal from emotional pain.

Thank you to my adoring and adorable family: Mom, Dad, Ben, Brinnon, Derek, Sophie, and Siena. Mom—thank you for the countless hours you spent on the phone with me during COVID debating whether I should use a comma or a semicolon, or start a fresh sentence. You seemingly have a Roget's *Thesaurus* on hand at all hours of the day and night when I'm stumped on a word that just isn't quite right. Thank you for continuing to snuggle with me, your now fortysomething-year-old adult child, and filling me with the warmth of your heart, always. Thank you to my dad for pulling out all the stops to try to keep me safe, comfortable, and very well fed. And thank you, Dad, for letting your feelings flow and for weeping with me in my pain and joy.

My true love, Derek. Thank you for loving me, in all my many versions, over the past twenty years. This book is a testament to my love for you that started so long ago at our college's local bar, when life was breezy and ripe with possibility. I'm so grateful that we chose one another, and I do not take for granted that you are standing firmly beside me, still brightening my world with your uproarious laughter, brilliant mind, and devoted, kind heart. Thank you for whooping and jumping up and down with me that night on West Seventieth Street when we learned about the book deal, and all the other innumerable ways you have championed me and the writing of our story. I love you madly and always will.

My sparkling Siena and Sophie, this book is for both of you. May it always remind you that my love for you is *unerasable*, a phrase I'm borrowing from Sophie. You two fill me with more delight and contentment than I could ever have possibly imagined.

Are you considering whether to transition from a narrative reader to a narrative writer? I applaud you! If your story includes a history of trauma, I strongly advise that you put pen to paper *after* establishing a supportive therapy relationship. Many traumas are interpersonal in nature (for instance, sexual assault or witnessing atrocities of war), and the reestablishment of trust and intimacy is central to recovery. The experience of a healthy, caring, and autonomy-supporting relationship with a therapist equips patients with a sense of safety and confidence to ultimately complete the at-times daunting work of facing a traumatic past.

Though I did not complete my trauma narrative as a formal component of my personal therapy with my psychologist, I knew that she was at the ready to support me in my writing endeavor; if ever I was drowning in psychological distress, she was my life jacket. I also decided to write on my own because I was already equipped with the psychological tools I teach my clients before they embark upon a successful narrative experience, including: an understanding of trauma; a regular relaxation practice; emotional awareness and regulation skills; and the ability to challenge faulty thinking patterns. If you decide to write—as I hope you will—I highly recommend that you practice these psychologically grounding interventions prior to commencing the challenging work of narrating your traumatic past. Below, I will share with you how I work with my clients to prepare them for their narrative work, as adapted from the writings of psychologists Marylene Cloitre, Lisa Cohen, and Karestan Koenen.[1]

1. Psychoeducation

Psychological education demystifies diagnoses, symptoms, and other trauma-related information. Symptoms are often experienced as overwhelming and terrifying—it feels, to my patients, as if they are perpetually living through their trauma over and over again. The waking hours are filled with intrusive memories, emotional reactions, and highly distressing body sensations. The sleeping hours are marked by trauma-laden nightmares. To hear from an expert that *we know what you're feeling* and *what you're feeling makes sense* and *we know how to help you feel better* provides not only the validation that what they are experiencing is real, but also the hope that what they are feeling now is not how they will feel forever. Normalizing the patient's symptoms through naming—*this is what we see in response to trauma*—helps patients realize that they are not crazy and that they are not alone.

2. Diaphragmatic breathing

This involves deep, steady breathing that acts to calm the nervous system and give the brain the signal that the body is not in danger. Patients are then armed with a potent relaxation intervention that they can use wherever they are (in a work meeting, commuting, before going to sleep), as they always have their breath. Clients are instructed to practice deep breathing daily as a way not only to calm the body but also to be able to safely *feel* and *be* with the body—a behavior that may have been avoided up to now because looking inward, to sensations, could have been triggering. Diaphragmatic breathing offers a way to gently exert control over a body that has felt out of control.

3. Naming and regulating emotions

Many people struggle with *alexithymia*, which refers to difficulty recognizing and describing one's own feelings. Combined with emotional detachment, which often presents itself with trauma, identification of emotion states can feel like trying to grab a fish in the ocean—there are glimpses of feelings, but they seemingly slip away. So collaboratively, we identify situations in which the patient has felt any distressing emotion and break down this elusive task into its component parts. *What thoughts were coming up at the time* ("If I'm vulnerable then I'll be taken advantage of ")? *What did you feel in your body* (heart racing, dizziness, abdominal distress)? *What did you do, behaviorally* (stay in bed all day, smoke pot to numb out)? *What were you feeling* (expanding upon the patients' perhaps limited emotional repertoire of "upset" to include rage, terror, jealousy)?

Emotion regulation includes emotional awareness and the ability to modulate, or adjust, feelings. Patients learn that they can increase positive emotions in their daily life by engaging in activities that they once enjoyed. I teach my clients emotional grounding exercises such as scanning a room and naming objects, or counting backward from 100 by 7s. As is the case throughout the therapy, patients practice the exercises they learn in session as homework between sessions in order to generalize the learning to everyday life.

4. Revising relationship patterns and beliefs

This is an opportunity for the client to challenge trauma-based cognitions that were likely adaptive during the crisis days of the past but are no longer adaptive in the safety of the present. The client revises interpersonal expectations, learns assertiveness techniques, and practices them in live role-plays with me during sessions.

A therapist with expertise in trauma treatment can help you master the above techniques, give you a sense of greater control and competence, and guide you through the writing of your trauma narrative, skillfully. You can find a therapist by visiting the Resources section of this appendix, which will direct you to websites where you can search for trauma-specialized providers. Traveling alongside you on your writing path, your therapist will bear witness and provide gentle direction if you feel lost.

RESOURCES

FOR IMMEDIATE SUPPORT

The National Suicide Prevention Lifeline
800-273-TALK (800-273-8255)
Available 24 hours in English and Spanish
www.suicidepreventionlifeline.org

Suicide Prevention Hotline
1-800-SUICIDE (800-784-2433)

The Crisis Text Line
Text HOME to 741741

PSYCHOTHERAPY-RELATED RESOURCES

Psychology Today, https://www.psychologytoday.com/us

Association for Behavioral and Cognitive Therapies, https://www.find
cbt.org/FAT/

Anxiety Disorders Association of America, www.adaa.org

American Psychological Association, www.apa.org

American Psychiatric Association, https://www.psychiatry.org/patients
-families

Ask for a therapy referral from your primary care provider.

Contact local hospitals and academic centers to find out if they offer psychotherapy services.

TRAUMA-RELATED SUPPORT AND RESOURCES
Websites

National Institute of Mental Health, www.nimh.nih.gov/health/topics
/post-traumatic-stress-disorder-ptsd

PTSD Alliance, www.ptsdalliance.org

Books

The Body Keeps the Score: Brain, Mind, and Body in the Healing of Trauma,
by Bessel van der Kolk, M.D.

*Trauma and Recovery: The Aftermath of Violence—from Domestic Abuse to
Political Terror*, by Judith Herman, M.D.

Get Out of Your Mind and Into Your Life, by Steven C. Hayes, Ph.D.
(This workbook is especially recommended for managing anxiety and
uncertainty with mindfulness-based interventions.)

CANCER-RELATED INFORMATION AND SUPPORT
Websites and Helplines

Memorial Sloan Kettering, www.mskcc.org

Dana Farber Institute, www.dana-farber.org

MD Anderson Cancer Center, www.mdanderson.org

Susan G. Komen Breast Care Helpline: 1-877-GO KOMEN (877-465-6636), www.komen.org

Young Survival Coalition, www.youngsurvival.org
For young women with breast cancer.

MATERNAL MENTAL HEALTH SUPPORT
Websites and Helplines

Postpartum Support International, www.postpartum.net
Helpline in English and Spanish: 800-944-4PPD (800-994-4773)
Text support: English—HELP to 800-944-4773; Spanish—971-203-7773

The Motherhood Center, www.themotherhoodcenter.com

Books

The Pregnancy and Postpartum Anxiety Workbook: Practical Skills to Help You Overcome Anxiety, Worry, Panic Attacks, Obsessions, and Compulsions, by Pamela S. Wiegartz, Ph.D., and Kevin L. Gyoerkoe, Psy.D.

This Isn't What I Expected: Overcoming Postpartum Depression, by Karen R. Kleiman, MSW, LCSW, and Valerie Davis Raskin, M.D.

What No One Tells You: A Guide to Your Emotions from Pregnancy to Motherhood, by Alexandra Sacks, M.D., and Catherine Birndorf, M.D.

Operating Instructions, by Anne Lamott

NOTES

INTRODUCTION

1 American Cancer Society. (2019). *Breast Cancer: Facts & Figures 2019–2020.* Atlanta: American Cancer Society, Inc.

2 Baselga, J., J. Cortés, S.-B. Kim, S.-A. Im, R. Hegg, Y.-H. Im, L. Roman, J. L. Pedrini, T. Pienkowski, A. Knott, E. Clark, M. C. Benyunes, G. Ross, S. M. Swain. (2012). "Pertuzumab plus Trastuzumab plus Docetaxel for Metastatic Breast Cancer." *New England Journal of Medicine* 366 (2): 109–19.

3 American Psychiatric Association. (2013). *Diagnostic and Statistical Manual of Mental Disorders,* 5th ed. Arlington, VA: American Psychiatric Association.

4 Zayfert, C., C. B. Becker. (2007). *Cognitive-Behavioral Therapy for PTSD: A Case Formulation Approach.* New York: The Guilford Press.

5 Breedlove, S. M., M. R. Rosenzweig, N. V. Watson. (2007). *Biological Psychology: An Introduction to Behavioral, Cognitive, and Clinical Neuroscience,* 5th ed. Sunderland, MA: Sinauer Associates, Inc.

6 Craske, M. G., D. H. Barlow. (2008). "Panic Disorder and Agoraphobia." In *Clinical Handbook of Psychological Disorders*, 4th ed., edited by D. H. Barlow, 1–64. New York: The Guilford Press.

7 Foa, E. B., D. S. Riggs. (1994). "Posttraumatic Stress Disorder and Rape." In *Posttraumatic Stress Disorder: A Clinical Review*, edited by R. S. Pynoos, 133–63.

8 Cloitre, M., L. R. Cohen, K. C. Koenen. (2006). *Treating Survivors*

of Childhood Abuse: Psychotherapy for the Interrupted Life. New York: The Guilford Press.

9   Kilpatrick, D. G., H. S. Resnick, M. E. Milanak, M. W. Miller, K. M. Keyes, M. J. Friedman. (2013). "National Estimates of Exposure to Traumatic Events and PTSD Prevalence Using DSM-IV and DSM-V Criteria." *Journal of Traumatic Stress* 26 (5): 537–47.

10   Wegner, D. M., D. J. Schneider, S. R. Carter III, T. L. White. (1987). "Paradoxical Effects of Thought Suppression." *Journal of Personality and Social Psychology* 53 (1): 5–13.

11   Resick, P. A., C. M. Monson, S. L. Rizvi. (2008). "Posttraumatic Stress Disorder." In *Clinical Handbook of Psychological Disorders*, 4th ed., edited by D. H. Barlow, 65–122. New York: The Guilford Press.

12   Breedlove, S. M., M. R. Rosenzweig, N. V. Watson. (2007). *Biological Psychology: An Introduction to Behavioral, Cognitive, and Clinical Neuroscience*, 5th ed. Sunderland, MA: Sinauer Associates, Inc.

CHAPTER 1: A DIFFERENT PREGNANCY

1   Kleiman, K. (2005). *What Am I Thinking: Having a Baby after Postpartum Depression?* Bloomington, IN: Xlibris.

2   Josefsson, A., L. Angelsiöö, G. Berg, C. M. Ekström, C. Gunnervik, C. Nordin, G. Sydsjö. (2002). "Obstetric, Somatic, and Demographic Risk Factors for Postpartum Depressive Symptoms." *Obstetrics and Gynecology* 99 (2): 223–28.

3   Josefsson, A., et al. (2002).

4   Stone, S. D., A. E. Menken. (2008). *Perinatal and Postpartum Mood Disorders: Perspectives and Treatment Guide for the Health Care Practitioner.* New York: Springer.

CHAPTER 5: TIME TO TELL SOPHIE

1   Hadhazy, A. (2016). "How It's Possible for an Ordinary Person to Lift a Car." BBC.com. Accessed September 16, 2020. https://www.bbc.com/future/article/20160501-how-its-possible-for-an-ordinary-person-to-lift-a-car.

2   Cannon, W. B. (1915). *Bodily Changes in Pain, Hunger, Fear and Rage.* New York: D. Appleton & Company.

3   Zayfert, C., C. B. Becker. (2007). *Cognitive-Behavioral Therapy for PTSD: A Case Formulation Approach.* New York: The Guilford Press.

4   Zayfert, C., C. B. Becker. (2007).

5   Finn, D. (2017). "The Impact of Stress on Pain: Considerable Over-
     lap in the Neural Substrates and Circuitries of Stress and Pain." *Phys-
     iology News Magazine* 108: 25–27.

CHAPTER 6: HAIR

1   Memorial Sloan Kettering Cancer Center. (2021). "How Effective
     Is Scalp Cooling? Could I Still Lose My Hair?" Accessed March 26,
     2021. https://www.mskcc.org/cancer-care/patient-education/man
     aging-hair-loss-scalp-cooling.

CHAPTER 8: LEOPARD

1   Swain, S. M., J. Baselga, S.-B. Kim, J. Ro, V. Semiglazov, M. Cam-
     pone, E. Ciruelos, J.-M. Ferrero, A. Schneeweiss, S. Heeson, E. Clark,
     G. Ross, M. C. Benyunes, J. Cortés. (2015). "Pertuzumab, Trastu-
     zumab, and Docetaxel in HER2-Positive Metastatic Breast Cancer."
     New England Journal of Medicine 372 (8): 725.
2   Baselga, J., et al. (2012) "Pertuzumab plus Trastuzumab plus Doce-
     taxel for Metastatic Breast Cancer."

CHAPTER 10: THE FIRST DRIP

1   Weiss, R. B., R. C. Donehower, P. H. Wiernik, T. Ohnuma, R. J.
     Gralla, D. L. Trump, J. R. Baker, D. A. Van Echo, D. D. Von Hoff,
     B. Leyland-Jones. (1990). "Hypersensitivity Reactions from Taxol."
     Journal of Clinical Oncology 8 (7): 1263–268.

CHAPTER 11: ARE YOU MY CANCER?

1   Breastcancer.org. (2018). *Risk of Developing Breast Cancer.* Accessed
     April 4, 2021. https://www.breastcancer.org/symptoms/understand
     _bc/risk/understanding.
2   Keyser, E. A., B. C. Staat, M. B. Fausett, A. D. Shields. (2012).
     "Pregnancy-Associated Breast Cancer." *Obstetrics and Gynecology* 5
     (2): 94–99.
3   Metastatic Breast Cancer Network. (2019). "Incidence and Incidence
     Rates." Accessed April 2, 2021. http://mbcn.org/incidence-and-in
     cidence-rates/.
4   Kabat-Zinn, J. (2003). "Mindfulness-Based Interventions in Context:
     Past, Present, and Future." *Clinical Psychology Science and Practice* 10
     (2): 144–56.

CHAPTER 15: AN UNWANTED BODY

1 Foa, E. B., D. S. Riggs. (1994). "Posttraumatic Stress Disorder and Rape."

2 Herman, J. L. (2002). "Recovery from Psychological Trauma." *Psychiatry and Clinical Neurosciences* 52 (S1): S98–S103.

3 American Psychiatric Association. (2013). *Diagnostic and Statistical Manual of Mental Disorders*, 5th ed.

CHAPTER 16: GANESHA AND OTHER TRAUMA TRIGGERS

1 Resick, P. A., C. M. Monson, S. L. Rizvi. (2008). "Posttraumatic Stress Disorder."

2 Resick, P. A., C. M. Monson, S. L. Rizvi. (2008). "Posttraumatic Stress Disorder."

CHAPTER 18: MY FAVORITE NAME IS NED

1 Herman, J. (1992, 1997, 2015). *Trauma and Recovery: The Aftermath of Violence—from Domestic Abuse to Political Terror*. New York: Basic Books.

2 van der Kolk, B. A. (2003). "Posttraumatic Stress Disorder and the Nature of Trauma." In *Healing Trauma: Attachment, Mind, Body and Brain*, edited by M. F. Solomon and D. J. Siegel, New York: W. W. Norton and Company, 168–95.

3 van der Kolk, B. A. (2003). "Posttraumatic Stress Disorder and the Nature of Trauma."

4 DePrince, A. P., J. J. Freyd. (2007). "Trauma-Induced Dissociation." In *Handbook of PTSD: Science and Practice*, edited by M. J. Friedman, M. J. Keane, and P. A. Resick. New York: The Guilford Press, 135–50.

5 Herman, J. (1992, 1997, 2015). *Trauma and Recovery*.

6 van der Kolk, B. A. (2003). "Posttraumatic Stress Disorder and the Nature of Trauma."

7 Baselga, J., et al. "Pertuzumab plus Trastuzumab plus Docetaxel for Metastatic Breast Cancer."

CHAPTER 19: BUZZ OFF

1 Leahy, R. L., S. J. Holland. (2000). *Treatment Plans and Interventions for Depression and Anxiety Disorders*. New York: The Guilford Press.

2 Resick, P. A., C. M. Monson, S. L. Rizvi. (2008). "Posttraumatic Stress Disorder."

3   Kohlberg, L. (1966). "A Cognitive-Developmental Analysis of Children's Sex-Role Concepts and Attitudes." In *The Development of Sex Differences*, edited by E. E. Maccoby. Stanford, CA: Stanford University Press, 82–173.

4   Omotoso, S. A. (2018). "Gender and Hair Politics: An African Philosophical Analysis." *Africology: The Journal of Pan African Studies* 12 (8): 5–19.

5   American Psychological Association. (2014). *Transgender People, Gender Identity and Gender Expression*. Accessed April 6, 2021. https://www.apa.org/topics/lgbtq/transgender.

CHAPTER 20: IN THE HAZE

1   Janelsins, M.C., C. E. Heckler, L. J. Peppone, C. Kamen, K. M. Mustian, S. G. Mohile, A. Magnuson, I. R. Kleckner, J. J. Guido, K. L. Young, A. K. Conlin, L. R. Weiselberg, J. W. Mitchell, C. A. Ambrosone, T. A. Ahles, G. R. Morrow. (2016). "Cognitive Complaints in Survivors of Breast Cancer after Chemotherapy Compared with Age-Matched Controls: An Analysis from a Nationwide, Multicenter, Prospective Longitudinal Study." *Journal of Clinical Oncology* 35 (5): 506–14.

2   Dornelas, E. A. (2018). *Psychological Treatment of Patients with Cancer*. Washington, DC: American Psychological Association.

3   Dornelas, E. A. (2018). *Psychological Treatment of Patients with Cancer*.

4   Collins, B. (2001). "Forgetfulness." In *Sailing Alone Around the Room: New and Selected Poems*. New York: Random House, 29.

CHAPTER 21: THE MIRROR

1   Cloitre, M., L. R. Cohen, K. C. Koenen. (2006). *Treating Survivors of Childhood Abuse*.

2   van der Kolk, B. A. (2014). *The Body Keeps the Score: Brain, Mind, and Body in the Healing of Trauma*. New York: Penguin.

3   Herman, J. (1992, 1997, 2015). *Trauma and Recovery*.

4   Herman, J. (1992, 1997, 2015). *Trauma and Recovery*. Quotations, 42–43.

5   Levine, P. A. (1997). *Waking the Tiger: Healing Trauma*. Berkeley, CA: North Atlantic Books.

6   Levine, P. A. (1997). *Waking the Tiger*.

7   Schore, A. N. (2003). "Early Relational Trauma, Disorganized Attachment, and the Development of a Predisposition to Violence." In

Healing Trauma: Attachment, Mind, Body and Brain, edited by M. F. Solomon and D. J. Siegel. New York: W. W. Norton and Company, 107–167.

8   Herman, J. (1992, 1997, 2015). *Trauma and Recovery.*

9   Levine, P. A. (1997). *Waking the Tiger.*

10   van der Kolk, B. A. (2014). *The Body Keeps the Score.*

11   Cloitre, M., L. R. Cohen, K. C. Koenen. (2006). *Treating Survivors of Childhood Abuse.*

CHAPTER 23: PAST MEETS PRESENT

1   van der Kolk, B. A. (2002). "Trauma and Memory." *Psychiatry and Clinical Neurosciences* 52 (51): 52–64.

CHAPTER 24: MOVING TOWARD RECOVERY

1   van der Kolk, B. A. (2014). *The Body Keeps the Score.*

2   Steele, K., O. van der Hart. (2009). "Treating Dissociation." In *Treating Complex Traumatic Stress Disorders: An Evidence-Based Guide,* edited by C. A. Courtois and J. D. Ford. New York: The Guilford Press, 145–65.

3   Levine, P. A. (1997). *Waking the Tiger.*

CHAPTER 25: CANCER-INDUCED ADOLESCENCE

1   Killingsworth, M. A., D. T. Gilbert. (2010). "A Wandering Mind Is an Unhappy Mind." *Science* 330 (6006): 932.

CHAPTER 26: RETURN FROM MATERNITY LEAVE

1   Breedlove, M. S., M. R. Rosenzweig, N. V. Watson. (2007). *Biological Psychology: An Introduction to Behavioral, Cognitive, and Clinical Neuroscience,* 5th ed. New York: Oxford University Press.

2   Pillai, J. A., C. B. Hall, D. W. Dickson, H. Buschke, R. B. Lipton, J. Verghese. (2011). "Association of Crossword Puzzle Participation with Memory Decline in Persons Who Develop Dementia." *Journal of the International Neuropsychological Society* 17 (6): 1006–1013.

3   Kunst, J. (2012). "Transference 101: Why a Blank Screen and Not a Real Person? How the Strange Method Is for Real." Psychology Today.com. Accessed April 12, 2021. https://www.psychology today.com/us/blog/headshrinkers-guide-the-galaxy/201203 /transference-101-why-blank-screen-and-not-real-person.

4   American Cancer Society. (2019). *Breast Cancer: Facts & Figures 2019–2020.* Atlanta, Georgia.

CHAPTER 27: FUNERAL MUSINGS

1   van der Kolk, B. A. (2003). "Posttraumatic Stress Disorder and the Nature of Trauma."
2   Dornelas, E. A. (2018). *Psychological Treatment of Patients with Cancer.*

CHAPTER 28: A TWISTED SPINE

1   Ogden, P., K. Minton, C. Pain. (2006). *Trauma and the Body: A Sensorimotor Approach to Psychotherapy.* New York: W. W. Norton & Company.
2   van der Kolk, B. A. (2003). "Posttraumatic Stress Disorder and the Nature of Trauma."
3   Fisher, J., P. Odgen. (2009). "Sensorimotor Psychotherapy." In *Treating Complex Traumatic Stress Disorders: An Evidence-Based Guide,* edited by C. A. Courtois and J. D. Ford. New York: The Guilford Press, 312–28.
4   Levine, P. A. (1997). *Waking the Tiger.*
5   Ogden, P., K. Minton, C. Pain. (2006). *Trauma and the Body,* 187.
6   Levine, P. A. (1997). *Waking the Tiger,* 38.
7   Ogden, P., K. Minton, C. Pain. (2006). *Trauma and the Body,* 227.
8   Ogden, P., K. Minton, C. Pain. (2006). *Trauma and the Body.*
9   van der Kolk, B. A., L. Stone, J. West, A. Rhodes, D. Emerson, M. Suvak, J. Spinazzola. (2014). "Yoga as an Adjunctive Treatment for Posttraumatic Stress Disorder: A Randomized Controlled Trial." *Journal of Clinical Psychiatry* 75 (6): 559–65.

CHAPTER 30: HISTORY CAN'T GUIDE US

1   Baselga, J., et al. (2012). "Pertuzumab plus Trastuzumab plus Docetaxel for Metastatic Breast Cancer."
2   Temple, S. (2017). *Brief Cognitive Behavior Therapy for Cancer Patients: Re-Visioning the CBT Paradigm.* New York: Routledge.
3   Dornelas, E. A. (2018). *Psychological Treatment of Patients with Cancer.*

CHAPTER 31: TABLE 5

1   Herman, J. (1992, 1997, 2015). *Trauma and Recovery.*

CHAPTER 32: LIVING IN IT

1   Woolf, V. (1930). *On Being Ill*. London: The Hogarth Press.

CHAPTER 37: INFORMED DENIAL

1   Dornelas, E. A. (2018). *Psychological Treatment of Patients with Cancer*.
2   Smith, H. R. (2015). "Depression in Cancer Patients: Pathogenesis,
     Implications, and Treatment" (Review). *Oncology Letters* 9: 1509–514.
3   Moreno-Smith, M., S. K. Lutgendorf, A. K. Sood. (2010). "Impact of
     Stress on Cancer Metastasis." *Future Oncology* 6 (12): 1863–881.
4   Dornelas, E. A. (2018). *Psychological Treatment of Patients with Cancer*.
5   Levine, M., D. D. Perkins, D. V. Perkins. (2005). *Principles of Commu-
     nity Psychology*, 3rd ed. New York: Oxford University Press.
6   Alizadeh, S., S. Khanahmadi, A. Vedadhir, S. Barjasteh. (2018). "The
     Relationship Between Resilience with Self-Compassion, Social Sup-
     port and Sense of Belonging in Women with Breast Cancer." *Asian
     Pacific Journal of Cancer Prevention* 19 (9): 2469–474.
7   McCann, L., L. A. Pearlman. (1990). "Vicarious Traumatization: A
     Framework for Understanding the Psychological Effects of Work-
     ing with Victims." *Journal of Traumatic Stress* 3 (1): 131–49.

CHAPTER 38: WHAT'S NEXT

1   Siegel, D. (2003). "An Interpersonal Neurobiology of Psychother-
     apy: The Developing Mind and the Resolution of Trauma." In *Heal-
     ing Trauma: Attachment, Mind, Body and Brain*, edited by M. Solomon
     and D. Siegel. New York: W. W. Norton & Company, 1–56.
2   van der Kolk, B. A. (2002). "Trauma and Memory."
3   Cloitre, M., L. R. Cohen, K. C. Koenen. (2006). *Treating Survivors of
     Childhood Abuse*.
4   Herman, J. (1992, 1997, 2015). *Trauma and Recovery*. Quotation from
     Sylvia Fraser, 213.

CHAPTER 39: THE OTHER BIG C

1   Cloitre, M., L. R. Cohen, K. C. Koenen. (2006). *Treating Survivors of
     Childhood Abuse*.

CHAPTER 42: LITTLE EARTHQUAKES

1   Fuller, T., A. Singhvi, M. Gröndahl, D. Watkins. (2019). "Buildings
     Can Be Designed to Withstand Earthquakes. Why Doesn't the U.S.

Build More of Them?" nytimes.com. Accessed December 22, 2020. https://www.nytimes.com/interactive/2019/06/03/us/earthquake -preparedness-usa-japan.html.

EPILOGUE

1   Gould, S. J. (1983). "The Median Isn't the Message." *Discover Magazine*. June 6: 40–42.
2   Solnit, R. (2013). *The Faraway Nearby*. New York: Penguin, 193.

A GUIDE TO NARRATIVE THERAPY

1   Cloitre, M., L. R. Cohen, K. C. Koenen. (2006). *Treating Survivors of Childhood Abuse*.
2   Herman, J. (1992, 1997, 2015). *Trauma and Recovery*. Quotation from Sylvia Fraser, 213.

ABOUT THE AUTHOR

SARAH MANDEL is a clinical psychologist. She lives in Manhattan with her husband and two daughters.